Gastroenterology for the Internist

Editor

KERRY B. DUNBAR

MEDICAL CLINICS
OF NORTH AMERICA

www.medical.theclinics.com

Consulting Editor
BIMAL H. ASHAR

January 2019 • Volume 103 • Number 1

ELSEVIER

1600 John F. Kennedy Boulevard • Suite 1800 • Philadelphia, Pennsylvania, 19103-2899

http://www.theclinics.com

MEDICAL CLINICS OF NORTH AMERICA Volume 103, Number 1
January 2019 ISSN 0025-7125, ISBN-13: 978-0-323-65469-2

Editor: Jessica McCool
Developmental Editor: Kristen Helm

Medical Clinics of North America (ISSN 0025-7125) is published bimonthly by Elsevier Inc., 360 Park Avenue South, New York, NY 10010-1710. Months of publication are January, March, May, July, September, and November. Business and editorial offices: 1600 John F. Kennedy Boulevard, Suite 1800, Philadelphia, PA 19103-2899. Periodicals postage paid at New York, NY, and additional mailing offices. Subscription prices are USD $284.00 per year (US individuals), $611.00 per year (US institutions), $100.00 per year (US Students), $353.00 per year (Canadian individuals), $794.00 per year (Canadian institutions), $200.00 per year (Canadian and foreign students), $406.00 per year (foreign individuals), and $794.00 per year (foreign institutions). To receive student/resident rate, orders must be accompanied by name of affiliated institution, date of term, and the signature of program/residency coordinator on institution letterhead. Orders will be billed at individual rate until proof of status is received. Foreign air speed delivery is included in all Clinics' subscription prices. All prices are subject to change without notice. **POSTMASTER:** Send address changes to *Medical Clinics of North America*, Elsevier Health Sciences Division, Subscription Customer Service, 3251 Riverport Lane, Maryland Heights, MO 63043. **Customer Service: Telephone: 1-800-654-2452** (U.S. and Canada); **1-314-447-8871** (outside U.S. and Canada). **Fax: 314-447-8029. E-mail: journalscustomerserviceusa@elsevier.com** (for print support); **journalsonlinesupport-usa@elsevier.com** (for online support).

Reprints. For copies of 100 or more of articles in this publication, please contact the Commercial Reprints Department, Elsevier Inc., 360 Park Avenue South, New York, NY 10010-1710. Tel.: 212-633-3874; Fax: 212-633-3820; E-mail: reprints@elsevier.com.

Medical Clinics of North America is also published in Spanish by McGraw-Hill Interamericana Editores S. A., P.O. Box 5-237, 06500 Mexico, D.F., Mexico.

Medical Clinics of North America is covered in *MEDLINE/PubMed (Index Medicus), Current Contents, ASCA, Excerpta Medica, Science Citation Index,* and *ISI/BIOMED*.

PROGRAM OBJECTIVE

The goal of the *Medical Clinics of North America* is to keep practicing physicians up to date with current clinical practice by providing timely articles reviewing the state of the art in patient care.

TARGET AUDIENCE

All practicing physicians and other healthcare professionals.

LEARNING OBJECTIVES

Upon completion of this activity, participants will be able to:

1. Review the role of food and dietary recommendations in common gastrointestinal and liver diseases
2. Discuss diagnosis and treatment options for gastroparesis
3. Recognize clinical features and epidemiology of eosinophilic esophagitis.

ACCREDITATION

The Elsevier Office of Continuing Medical Education (EOCME) is accredited by the Accreditation Council for Continuing Medical Education (ACCME) to provide continuing medical education for physicians.

The EOCME designates this enduring material for a maximum of 15 *AMA PRA Category 1 Credit*(s)™. Physicians should claim only the credit commensurate with the extent of their participation in the activity.

All other healthcare professionals requesting continuing education credit for this enduring material will be issued a certificate of participation.

DISCLOSURE OF CONFLICTS OF INTEREST

The EOCME assesses conflict of interest with its instructors, faculty, planners, and other individuals who are in a position to control the content of CME activities. All relevant conflicts of interest that are identified are thoroughly vetted by EOCME for fair balance, scientific objectivity, and patient care recommendations. EOCME is committed to providing its learners with CME activities that promote improvements or quality in healthcare and not a specific proprietary business or a commercial interest.

The planning committee, staff, authors and editors listed below have identified no financial relationships or relationships to products or devices they or their spouse/life partner have with commercial interest related to the content of this CME activity:

Oviea Akpotaire, MD; Nuha Alammar, MD; Olaya I. Brewer Gutierrez, MD; Lisa Casey, MD; John O. Clarke, MD; Kelli DeLay, MD; Evan S. Dellon, MD, MPH; Jason A. Dominitz, MD, MHS; Kerry B. Dunbar, MD, PhD; Linda A. Feagins, MD; Alison Kemp; Anne Marie Lennon, MD, PhD; Peter S. Liang, MD, MPH; Khurram Mazhar, MD; Jessica McCool; Frances U. Onyimba, MD; Vaishali Patel, MD, MHS; Michelle Pearlman, MD; Craig C. Reed, MD; Ellen Stein, MD; Jeyanthi Surendrakumar; Alison Swety; Field Willingham, MD, MPH, FASGE.

The planning committee, staff, authors and editors listed below have identified financial relationships or relationships to products or devices they or their spouse/life partner have with commercial interest related to the content of this CME activity:

William M. Lee, MD: is a consultant/advisor for Genentech, Inc., Novartis AG, and Sanofi and receives research support from Conatus Pharmaceuticals, Inc., Gilead, and Intercept Pharmaceuticals, Inc.
Jordan Mayberry, PA-C: is a consultant/advisor for Dova Pharmaceuticals and is a consultant/advisor and participated on a speakers bureau for Gilead, AbbVie Inc. and Intercept Pharmaceuticals, Inc.
Stuart Jon Spechler, MD: is a consultant/advisor for Takeda Pharmaceuticals Company Limited and Ironwood Pharmaceuticals, Inc. and receives royalties from UpToDate, Inc.
Rena Yadlapati, MD, MSHS: is a consultant/advisor for Ironwood Pharmaceuticals, Inc., Medtronic, and Diversatek, Inc.

UNAPPROVED/OFF-LABEL USE DISCLOSURE

The EOCME requires CME faculty to disclose to the participants;

1. When products or procedures being discussed are off-label, unlabelled, experimental, and/or investigational (not US Food and Drug Administration [FDA] approved); and
2. Any limitations on the information presented, such as data that are preliminary or that represent ongoing research, interim analyses, and/or unsupported opinions. Faculty may discuss information about pharmaceutical agents that is outside of FDA-approved labelling. This information is intended solely for CME and is not intended to promote off-label use of these medications. If you have any questions, contact the medical affairs department of the manufacturer for the most recent prescribing information.

TO ENROLL

To enroll in the *Medical Clinics of North America* Continuing Medical Education program, call customer service at 1-800-654-2452 or sign up online at http://www.theclinics.com/home/cme. The CME program is available to subscribers for an additional annual fee of USD $300.90.

METHOD OF PARTICIPATION

In order to claim credit, participants must complete the following;
1. Complete enrolment as indicated above.
2. Read the activity.
3. Complete the CME Test and Evaluation. Participants must achieve a score of 70% on the test. All CME Tests and Evaluations must be completed online.

CME INQUIRIES/SPECIAL NEEDS

For all CME inquiries or special needs, please contact elsevierCME@elsevier.com.

MEDICAL CLINICS OF NORTH AMERICA

MEDICAL CLINICS OF NORTH AMERICA

FORTHCOMING ISSUES	RECENT ISSUES
November 2019	
Group ...	
C. Matthew Stewart, Editor	
September 2019	
Anticoagulation	
Geno J. Merli, Editor	
July 2019	
Substance Use and Addiction Medicine	
Jeffrey H. Samet, Patrick G. O'Connor, and	
Michael D. Stein, Editors	

ISSUE OF RELATED INTEREST

Primary Care: Clinics in Office Practice, December 2017 (Vol. 44, No. 4)
Gastroenterology
... Kellerman and Laurie Nunno, Editors
Available at: http://www.primarycare.theclinics.com

Contributors

CONSULTING EDITOR

BIMAL H. ASHAR, MD, MBA, FACP
Associate Professor of Medicine, Division of General Internal Medicine, Johns Hopkins University School of Medicine, Baltimore, Maryland, USA

EDITOR

KERRY B. DUNBAR, MD, PhD
Associate Professor of Medicine, Section Chief (VA), Gastroenterology, Dallas VA Medical Center-VA North Texas Healthcare System, Associate Program Director, Internal Medicine, University of Texas Southwestern Medical Center, Dallas, Texas, USA

AUTHORS

OVIEA AKPOTAIRE, MD
Department of Internal Medicine, University of Texas Southwestern, Dallas, Texas, USA

NUHA ALAMMAR, MD
Faculty, Department of Medicine, Division of Gastroenterology, King Khalid University Hospital, King Saud University, Riyadh, Saudi Arabia

OLAYA I. BREWER GUTIERREZ, MD
Division of Gastroenterology and Hepatology, Johns Hopkins Medical Institution, Advanced Therapeutic Fellow, The Johns Hopkins Hospital, Baltimore, Maryland, USA

LISA CASEY, MD
Assistant Professor, Department of Internal Medicine, Division of Digestive and Liver Diseases, University of Texas Southwestern, Dallas, Texas, USA

JOHN O. CLARKE, MD
Department of Medicine, Division of Gastroenterology and Hepatology, Stanford University, Stanford, California, USA

KELLI DeLAY, MD
Division of Gastroenterology and Hepatology, University of Colorado Anschutz Medical Campus, Aurora, Colorado, USA

EVAN S. DELLON, MD, MPH
Division of Gastroenterology and Hepatology, Department of Medicine, Center for Esophageal Diseases and Swallowing, Center for Gastrointestinal Biology and Disease, University of North Carolina School of Medicine, Chapel Hill, North Carolina, USA

JASON A. DOMINITZ, MD, MHS
Gastroenterology Section, VA Puget Sound Health Care System, Division of
Gastroenterology, Department of Medicine, University of Washington School of
Medicine, Seattle, Washington, USA

LINDA ANNE FEAGINS, MD
Division of Gastroenterology and Hepatology, Associate Professor of Medicine,
University of Texas Southwestern Medical Center, Staff Physician, VA North Texas
Healthcare System, Dallas VA Medical Center, Dallas, Texas, USA

WILLIAM M. LEE, MD
Meredith Mosle Chair in Liver Diseases, Professor of Internal Medicine, Division of
Digestive and Liver Diseases, University of Texas Southwestern Medical Center at Dallas,
Dallas, Texas, USA

ANNE MARIE LENNON, MD, PhD
Division of Gastroenterology and Hepatology, Associate Professor, Medicine, Surgery,
Oncology and Radiology, Clinical Director of Gastroenterology, Director, Multidisciplinary
Pancreatic Cyst Clinic, The Johns Hopkins Medical Institutions, Baltimore, Maryland, USA

PETER S. LIANG, MD, MPH
Gastroenterology Section, Department of Medicine, VA New York Harbor Health Care
System, Division of Gastroenterology, Department of Medicine, NYU Langone Health,
New York, New York, USA

JORDAN MAYBERRY, PA-C
Physician Assistant, Division of Digestive and Liver Diseases, University of Texas
Southwestern Medical Center at Dallas, Dallas, Texas, USA

KHURRAM MAZHAR, MD
Assistant Professor, Department of Internal Medicine, Division of Digestive and
Liver Diseases, University of Texas Southwestern Medical Center, North Texas VA
Health Care System, Division of Gastroenterology, Dallas VA Medical Center, Dallas,
Texas, USA

FRANCES U. ONYIMBA, MD
Department of Medicine, Division of Gastroenterology, University of California San Diego,
La Jolla, California, USA

VAISHALI PATEL, MD, MHS
Division of Digestive Diseases, Assistant Professor, Department of Medicine, Emory
University School of Medicine, Atlanta, Georgia, USA

MICHELLE PEARLMAN, MD
Physician Nutrition Specialist, Gastroenterology and Hepatology Fellow, Department of
Internal Medicine, Division of Digestive and Liver Diseases, University of Texas South-
western, Dallas, Texas, USA

CRAIG C. REED, MD, MSCR
Division of Gastroenterology and Hepatology, Department of Medicine, Center
for Esophageal Diseases and Swallowing, Center for Gastrointestinal Biology and
Disease, University of North Carolina School of Medicine, Chapel Hill, North Carolina,
USA

STUART JON SPECHLER, MD
Division of Gastroenterology, Center for Esophageal Diseases, Baylor University Medical Center, Center for Esophageal Research, Baylor Scott and White Research Institute, Dallas, Texas, USA

ELLEN STEIN, MD
Assistant Professor, Department of Medicine, Division of Gastroenterology, Johns Hopkins University, Baltimore, Maryland, USA

FIELD WILLINGHAM, MD, MPH, FASGE
Division of Digestive Diseases, Associate Professor, Department of Medicine, Director of Endoscopy, Emory University Hospital, Medical Director of Therapeutic Endoscopy, Children's Healthcare of Atlanta, Emory University School of Medicine, Atlanta, Georgia, USA

RENA YADLAPATI, MD, MSHS
Division of Gastroenterology and Hepatology, University of Colorado Anschutz Medical Campus, Aurora, Colorado, USA

Contents

This report reviews the physiology of gastric acid suppression by proton pump inhibitors (PPIs) and anti-inflammatory effects of PPIs that are independent of their acid-suppressive effects. Valid indications for PPI use are discussed, as are putative adverse effects of PPIs that have been identified through weak associations in observational studies that cannot establish cause-and-effect relationships. Although evidence supporting the validity of these adverse effects is weak, there is also insufficient evidence to dismiss the risks. The report emphasizes how PPIs frequently are prescribed inappropriately and encourages physicians to carefully consider the indication for PPI therapy in their patients.

Proton pump inhibitor (PPI)-refractory gastroesophageal reflux disease (GERD) is defined by the presence of troublesome GERD symptoms despite PPI optimization for at least 8 weeks in the setting of ongoing documented pathologic gastroesophageal reflux. It arises from a dysfunction in protective systems to prevent reflux and as propagation of physiologic reflux events. Treatment possibilities include pharmacologic options, invasive management strategies, and endoluminal therapies. Management strategy should be personalized to the patient's needs and mechanistic dysfunction. This article reviews the definition, mechanisms, and management options for PPI-refractory GERD.

Eosinophilic esophagitis (EoE) is a chronic disorder characterized by symptoms of esophageal dysfunction and esophageal inflammation with intraepithelial eosinophils. EoE represents an important cause of upper gastrointestinal morbidity. Primary care providers are pivotal for timely and accurate recognition of symptoms of eosinophilic esophagitis, for facilitating diagnoses through specialist referrals, and for understanding management strategies. This process begins with a thorough understanding of the clinical features of EoE, its associated atopic conditions, and its evolving epidemiology.

counsel their patients and minimize potential complications from following such a restrictive diet.

Food plays an essential role in normal cellular processes; however, certain foods may also trigger or worsen certain disease states. This article focuses particularly on the role of food in common gastrointestinal and liver diseases, and discusses the current evidence that either supports or debunks common dietary recommendations. Nutrition topics discussed include the use of artificial sweetener for weight loss, avoidance of all dairy products in the setting of lactose intolerance, dietary recommendations for diverticular disease, and dietary management in cirrhotic patients with hepatic encephalopathy.

Colorectal cancer is the second leading cause of cancer death in the United States. Prospective studies demonstrate that colorectal cancer screening reduces incidence and mortality, but uptake remains suboptimal. More than a third of age-eligible Americans are not up to date on screening. There are several available screening tests, which may cause primary care providers to ponder which is the best test. This article provides an overview of the available test options and the evidence for each; a summary of major guidelines; and a comparison of the two most widely used tests, colonoscopy and fecal immunochemical testing.

Colonoscopy with polypectomy is the means by which the incidence of colon cancer may be reduced; however, polypectomy is not without risk. Physicians must carefully weigh the risks and benefits of colonoscopy, particularly when patients are given prescriptions for antiplatelet agents and anticoagulants. This article discusses the risks of colonoscopy and polypectomy and reviews the most recent data for managing antiplatelet agents and anticoagulants in the periendoscopic period.

Irritable bowel syndrome (IBS) is present in patients with symptoms of chronic abdominal pain and altered bowel habits but no identifiable organic etiology. Rome IV classification groups patients based on predominant stool pattern. Low-FODMAP diets have been helpful in providing symptom relief, as have cognitive behavioral and mind-body techniques that help patients manage symptoms. Targeted symptomatic relief for the patient's predominant symptoms provides relief in addition to effective older medications that are inexpensive and reliable. Newer treatments for

Chronic pancreatitis (CP) may remain undiagnosed for years until patients exhibit manifestations, such as pain and exocrine or endocrine insufficiency. Some patients with CP develop serious complications, such as malignancy or peripancreatic fluid collections. Considering CP in at-risk patients such as those with a long-standing history of alcohol or tobacco use is key to establishing the diagnosis. Management involves reducing and eliminating exposures, dietary modification, treatment of pancreatic insufficiency, assessing for complications, and surveillance for neoplasia. The management of CP is often multidisciplinary involving medical, endoscopic, and surgical options for therapy.

Pancreatic cysts are common and are incidentally detected in up to 13.5% of individuals. Intraductal papillary mucinous neoplasm (IPMN) and mucinous cystic neoplasm (MCN) are precursors to pancreatic adenocarcinoma. Most will never develop into pancreatic cancer. Several types of pancreatic cysts have no malignant potential. Solid tumors can present as a pancreatic cysts. Guidelines recommend surveillance. Management includes differentiating IPMNs and MCNs from other types, identifying those at highest risk of harboring pancreatic cancer or high-grade dysplasia, and referral to a multidisciplinary group for evaluation and consideration of surgical resection.

Foreword
Gut Check

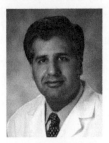

Bimal H. Ashar, MD, MBA, FACP
Consulting Editor

"All disease begins in the gut." This quote from Hippocrates may not be a scientifically proven fact, but it does underscore the importance of the gastrointestinal system for overall health. The relationship between the brain and the gut has made its way into the English language through slang and phrases. People get "butterflies in their stomach" when they are nervous. One may "bust a gut" when they are laughing hard, "hate someone's guts" when they are angry, and "go with their gut" when using their intuition. People are familiar with emotional situations triggering gastrointestinal symptoms. Yet, the reverse is also true: Gastrointestinal symptoms can also trigger anxiety, stress, or depression. Recently, I had a patient who suffered a diverticular bleed. He subsequently became so anxious about his bowel habits that he sent daily electronic messages for 2 months regarding the quantity, quality, and character of his bowel movements. Days without movements were even more anxiety-provoking, with the patient inquiring about medical intervention.

The importance of the gastrointestinal system in the development of other diseases is also undergoing extensive research. Alterations in the gut microbiome have been associated with diseases such as autism, Parkinson disease, multiple sclerosis, and schizophrenia. Although evidence to date is correlative and not causative, it is an exciting field of inquiry that it is hoped will allow for more holistic treatment of some disorders.

In this issue of *Medical Clinics of North America*, Dr Dunbar and her colleagues have not focused on the investigational but have chosen topics seen frequently in primary care practice. For example, gastroesophageal reflux disease affects nearly 60 million Americans, with about 15 million using proton pump inhibitors (PPIs) in some fashion. Dr Spechler delves into the controversies regarding PPIs in order to assist in developing the optimal treatment strategy for this common disorder. Dr Dunbar has also

Med Clin N Am 103 (2019) xv–xvi
https://doi.org/10.1016/j.mcna.2018.09.003
0025-7125/19/© 2018 Published by Elsevier Inc.

chosen to focus two articles of this issue on diet, emphasizing the importance of another of Hippocrates' beliefs: "Let food be thy medicine and medicine be thy food."

Bimal H. Ashar, MD, MBA, FACP
Division of General Internal Medicine
Johns Hopkins University School of Medicine
601 North Caroline Street
#7143
Baltimore, MD 21287, USA

E-mail address:
Bashar1@jhmi.edu

Preface

Gastroenterology for the Internist

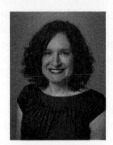

Kerry B. Dunbar, MD, PhD
Editor

Gastroenterology disorders such as gastroesophageal reflux disease (GERD) and irritable bowel syndrome are a common indication for primary care office visits. Patients with chronic gastroenterology and hepatology disorders are often followed closely by both internists and gastroenterologists. This issue of *Medical Clinics of North America* is dedicated to advances in the management of common gastroenterology and hepatology disorders managed by both internists and gastroenterologists and the new developments and challenges related to these disorders. Several of the articles address topics related to questions patients frequently ask, including proton pump inhibitors (PPI) safety, whether gluten-free diets are helpful, and common concerns about food. This issue also includes articles about management challenges seen by both internists and gastroenterologists, such as treatment of PPI-refractory GERD and evaluation of incidental pancreatic cysts. With an aging population, issues related to colorectal cancer screening are also frequently encountered in clinic practice, from choice of screening test to the management of anticoagulation and antiplatelet agents for colonoscopy. The incidence of liver disease is rising, and this issue includes updates about new advances in treatment of hepatitis C and management of nonalcoholic fatty liver disease. Guidance for other common gastrointestinal (GI) disorders, such as eosinophilic esophagitis, gastroparesis, chronic pancreatitis, and irritable bowel syndrome, is also included.

I would like to thank my distinguished colleagues for their outstanding contributions to this issue. On behalf of the authors, I hope you find this collection useful for current

Med Clin N Am 103 (2019) xvii–xviii
https://doi.org/10.1016/j.mcna.2018.09.002
0025-7125/19/© 2018 Published by Elsevier Inc.

clinical practice and future investigations into these common GI and hepatology topics.

Kerry B. Dunbar, MD, PhD
VA Gastroenterology Section
Dallas VA Medical Center–VA North Texas Healthcare System
Internal Medicine
University of Texas, Southwestern Medical Center
GI Lab, CA 111-B1, 4500 South Lancaster Road
Dallas, TX 75216, USA

E-mail addresses:
Kerry.Dunbar@va.gov
Kerry.Dunbar@utsouthwestern.edu

Proton Pump Inhibitors
What the Internist Needs to Know

Stuart Jon Spechler, MD

KEYWORDS

- Proton pump inhibitor • Complications • Peptic ulcer disease
- Gastroesophageal reflux disease

KEY POINTS

- Putative adverse effects of proton pump inhibitors (PPIs) have been identified through weak associations found in observational studies that cannot establish cause-and-effect relationships.
- Although evidence supporting the validity of putative adverse PPI effects generally is weak, there is also insufficient evidence to dismiss the risks entirely.
- PPIs frequently are prescribed inappropriately (for conditions unlikely to respond to PPI treatment) and often in higher-than-recommended dosages.
- Before prescribing PPIs, physicians should carefully consider whether the indication is valid and, if so, to confirm the appropriate dosing for the indication.
- For patients on PPIs, the physician should carefully review the medical record and determine whether continuation of PPI therapy is appropriate.

Proton pump inhibitors (PPIs) are among the most commonly used and overprescribed medications in the world.[1] In the United States alone, more than 7% of adults take prescription PPIs and, undoubtedly, many more use PPIs acquired over the counter.[2] These agents profoundly suppress gastric acid secretion, and they are widely regarded as the medications of choice for treating acid-peptic disorders, such as gastroesophageal reflux disease (GERD) and peptic ulcer disease. Well-established side effects of the PPIs, such as headache, diarrhea, constipation, and abdominal discomfort, are minor, relatively uncommon, and easily managed. Recent publications, however, describing numerous putative, serious PPI side effects have raised concern among patients and clinicians alike.

Conflict of Interest: S.J. Spechler has served as a consultant for Takeda Pharmaceuticals and Ironwood Pharmaceuticals, and receives royalties as an author for UpToDate.
Division of Gastroenterology, Center for Esophageal Diseases, Baylor University Medical Center, Center for Esophageal Research, Baylor Scott & White Research Institute, 3500 Gaston Avenue, 2 Hoblitzelle, Suite 250, Dallas, TX 75246, USA
E-mail address: sjspechler@aol.com

Med Clin N Am 103 (2019) 1–14
https://doi.org/10.1016/j.mcna.2018.08.001
0025-7125/19/© 2018 Elsevier Inc. All rights reserved.
medical.theclinics.com

INHIBITION OF GASTRIC ACID SECRETION BY PROTON PUMP INHIBITORS

Hydrochloric acid is secreted by parietal cells in the oxyntic mucosa that lines the body and fundus of the stomach. Parietal cells produce acid in response to 3 major stimuli:

1. Acetylcholine, which is released by some neurons that innervate the stomach
2. Histamine, which is produced by enterochromaffin-like (ECL) cells in the gastric oxyntic mucosa
3. Gastrin, which is secreted by endocrine G cells in the pyloric gland mucosa that lines the gastric antrum[3]

The parietal cell has a receptor for each of these molecules. Binding of acetylcholine to a subtype 3 muscarinic receptor on the parietal cell results in an increase in intracellular calcium (Ca^{2+}). Gastrin, which is a member of the same peptide hormone family as cholecystokinin (CCK), binds the parietal cell's CCK-2 receptor, which also causes an increase in intracellular Ca^{2+}. In addition, gastrin binds a CCK-2 receptor on gastric ECL cells, stimulating them to release histamine. This histamine binds to a histamine H_2 receptor on the parietal cell, activating adenylate cyclase to generate $3', 5'$-cyclic adenosine monophosphate (cAMP). Finally, the Ca^{2+} and cAMP induced by these stimulants activate H^+, K^+-ATPase, the proton pump of the parietal cell that pumps hydrogen ions (protons) into the lumen in exchange for potassium ions. PPIs block this final step in gastric acid secretion.

The PPIs available in the United States (omeprazole, esomeprazole, lansoprazole, dexlansoprazole, pantoprazole, and rabeprazole) are prodrugs that must be activated by acid to inhibit the proton pump.[4] Ironically, however, PPIs also are vulnerable to degradation by acid, and they are manufactured with an enteric coating that protects them from destruction by acid in the gastric lumen. When an ingested PPI is absorbed and transported through the blood to the secretory canaliculus of a parietal cell that is actively secreting acid, the weakly basic PPI molecule is protonated and concentrated in the parietal cell, where acid catalyzes conversion of the PPI prodrug to a reactive form called a sulfenamide. This sulfenamide binds covalently to cysteine residues on the luminal surface of the H^+, K^+-ATPase, irreversibly blocking its ability to secrete acid.

Because the PPIs are activated and bound only by proton pumps that are actively secreting acid, it is important to time PPI dosing around meals. In the fasting state, only approximately 5% of gastric proton pumps are active, whereas 60% to 70% of those proton pumps are active during a meal.[4] Thus, for maximal efficacy, PPIs should be taken 30 minutes to 60 minutes before a meal to allow time for the enteric-coated drug to be absorbed and available in the blood when the maximum number of proton pumps are susceptible to inhibition. For once-daily dosing, the PPIs should be taken 30 minutes to 60 minutes before breakfast. For twice-daily dosing, they should be taken 30 minutes to 60 minutes before breakfast and 30 minutes to 60minutes before dinner. Given in this fashion, PPIs are remarkably effective inhibitors of gastric acid secretion. PPIs do not eliminate gastric acid secretion entirely, however, especially at night. Approximately 70% to 80% of individuals treated with a PPI twice daily experience nocturnal gastric acid breakthrough, defined as a fall in gastric pH below 4 for more than 1 hour at night.[5] Nocturnal acid breakthrough does not necessarily cause symptoms or tissue damage nor does it seem to interfere with PPI-induced healing of acid-peptic disorders. Thus, the clinical importance of nocturnal gastric acid breakthrough is not clear.[6]

Among the available PPIs, dosing around meals is least critical for dexlansoprazole, which is marketed in a modified-release formulation that delivers the drug in 2 discrete phases.[7] The dexlansoprazole is contained in 2 types of granules that have different, pH-dependent dissolution profiles. One granule type releases the drug as soon as it reaches the mildly acidic duodenum, whereas the second granule type is designed to release the drug in the pH-neutral environment of the distal small bowel. This formulation gives dexlansoprazole a dual-peak time concentration profile. Although this provides some flexibility regarding dosing around meals, it is not clear that dexlansoprazole has any clinical advantage over other PPIs for healing acid-peptic diseases. The clinical efficacies of all the PPIs are approximately equal, although individual patients can exhibit considerable variability in the degree of acid suppression induced by different PPIs.[8]

Because PPIs are administered in forms that delay their release and absorption, after which they must be concentrated and activated within parietal cells, acid inhibition by PPIs is delayed for hours after dosing. Also, because a single meal does not activate all parietal cells and all of their proton pumps, it takes several days for PPIs to achieve their maximal effect on acid inhibition. Thus, although PPIs are the most effective long-term inhibitors of gastric acid secretion available in this country, acid inhibition by PPIs is not a rapid process. For the immediate relief of heartburn, an antacid or histamine H_2-receptor antagonist is a better choice than a PPI, even though the PPI is more effective than either of those agents for long-term relief of heartburn. There is also an immediate-release PPI preparation containing omeprazole with no enteric coating along with sodium bicarbonate, which neutralizes acid in the stomach lumen to prevent degradation of the acid-labile omeprazole.[9]

POTENTIAL ANTI-INFLAMMATORY EFFECTS OF PROTON PUMP INHIBITORS

In vitro studies have identified several potential anti-inflammatory effects of PPIs that are entirely independent of their effects on inhibiting gastric acid secretion.[10] For example, PPIs have antioxidant properties, including the ability to scavenge hydroxyl radicals,[11] to increase the bioavailability of sulfhydryl compounds that might raise glutathione levels,[12] and to induce heme oxygenase.[13] PPIs can suppress the oxidative burst of neutrophils and monocytes and can inhibit their ability to migrate and to phagocytose material.[14–18] PPIs also can inhibit the expression of certain cell adhesion molecules that are involved in the recruitment of inflammatory cells to sites of inflammation, including members of the CD11/CD18 integrin family, intercellular adhesion molecule 1, and vascular cell adhesion molecule 1.[17,19–21]

A clinical response to PPI treatment traditionally has been regarded as strong de facto evidence of acid-peptic disease with the rationale that suppression of gastric acid secretion is the only important effect of PPIs. This traditional concept has been challenged by increasing recognition of the potential importance of PPI anti-inflammatory effects. For patients with esophageal symptoms associated with esophageal eosinophilia, for example, a clinical response to PPIs had been regarded as evidence for GERD rather than eosinophilic esophagitis (EoE).[22] It now seems, however, that an anti-inflammatory action might underlie this beneficial effect of PPIs. In EoE, eosinophils accumulate in the esophageal mucosa when type 2 helper T-cell (T_H2) cytokines, such as interleukin (IL)-4 and IL-13, stimulate esophageal epithelial cells to secrete eotaxin-3, which is a potent eosinophil chemoattractant. Cheng and colleagues[23] used esophageal squamous cell lines to show that omeprazole can block the increase in eotaxin-3 mRNA expression and protein secretion stimulated by T_H2 cytokines. By blocking this cytokine-stimulated production of an eosinophil chemoattractant, PPIs might decrease esophageal eosinophilia in EoE. Thus, PPIs are now regarded as an EoE treatment rather than as a diagnostic test for GERD in patients with esophageal eosinophilia. Nevertheless, the precise contribution of PPI anti-inflammatory effects to their clinical benefits remains unclear.

VALID INDICATIONS FOR PROTON PUMP INHIBITOR USAGE

Box 1 lists the valid indications for PPI usage. For the conditions discussed in Box 1, there is general consensus that the benefits of PPIs clearly outweigh their potential risks.[24] The serious putative adverse effects of PPIs (discussed later) are associated predominantly with long-term usage. GERD is the most common valid indication for long-term PPI usage. Severe reflux esophagitis does not heal reliably with any available medication other than PPIs, and severe esophagitis returns quickly (within 1 week to 2 weeks) when PPIs are stopped.[25] Another valid and potentially life-saving indication for chronic PPI usage is to protect against peptic ulceration for patients taking nonsteroidal anti-inflammatory drugs (NSAIDs), who are at high risk for ulcer complications.[26] This includes patients with a history of peptic ulcer disease, patients age 65 years and older, and patients who concurrently use aspirin, steroids, or anticoagulants. Patients with EoE who respond to PPIs probably need to take PPIs indefinitely, and patients with rare hypersecretory conditions like Zollinger-Ellison syndrome also require long-term PPI treatment.

Several studies have documented that PPIs frequently are prescribed inappropriately, that is, for conditions unlikely to respond to PPI treatment.[1,27,28] For patients taking PPIs for any condition not listed in Box 1, the physician should carefully review the medical record and determine whether continuation of PPI therapy is appropriate. Such a review often reveals that PPIs should be discontinued.

PUTATIVE SERIOUS ADVERSE EFFECTS OF PROTON PUMP INHIBITOR THERAPY
Proton Pump Inhibitor Acid Suppression and Adverse Effects

Some of the putative adverse effects of PPIs are related to their profound suppression of gastric acid secretion. With such acid suppression, micro-organisms that would have been destroyed by gastric acid might colonize the upper gastrointestinal tract,

---

Box 1
Valid indications for proton pump inhibitor usage

Short-term treatment

Duodenal ulcer

Gastric ulcer

Helicobacter pylori eradication

Stress ulcer prophylaxis for critically ill patients with ulcer risk factors (respiratory failure, coagulopathy, head injury, extensive burns, acute hepatic failure, acute renal failure, hypotension, sepsis, or history of gastrointestinal bleeding)

Dyspepsia

Chronic treatment

GERD

NSAID ulcer prophylaxis in patients with ulcer risk factors (history of peptic ulcer, age ≥65 years, concomitant use of aspirin, steroids, or anticoagulants)

EoE

Hypersecretory conditions (Zollinger-Ellison syndrome)

---

thus altering its microbiome.[29] With PPIs blocking gastric acid production, furthermore, ingested microbial pathogens that otherwise would have been killed by gastric acid might survive and cause infections. Gastric acid inhibition by PPIs also can influence the uptake of certain vitamins (eg, vitamin B_{12}), minerals (eg, calcium and iron), and drugs (eg, ketoconazole and digoxin) whose absorption is affected by gastric acid.

Elevation of serum gastrin levels is another potentially undesirable effect of gastric acid suppression by PPIs. As discussed previously, gastrin released by G cells in the pyloric gland mucosa of the antrum stimulates acid secretion by parietal cells in the gastric body and fundus. When that acid reaches the antrum, it activates a neuronal reflex that stimulates endocrine D cells in the pyloric gland mucosa to produce somatostatin.[3] This somatostatin inhibits the release of gastrin from the adjacent G cells, thereby turning off parietal cell acid secretion. When PPIs block production of the acid needed to turn off gastrin production, gastrin secretion continues unabated and serum gastrin levels rise.[30] Gastrin is a growth factor that can increase proliferation in ECL cells, in Barrett metaplasia and in the colon.[31–33] Chronic PPI treatment has been found to elevate serum levels of chromogranin A, an index of ECL cell mass.[33] Increased ECL cell mass has been proposed to explain the phenomenon of "rebound acid hypersecretion" in which abrupt termination of chronic PPI therapy results in levels of gastric acid production exceeding those measured before PPI treatment.[34] This rebound acid hypersecretion can persist for months after the termination of chronic PPI therapy, but its clinical importance remains unclear.

General Categories of Proposed proton Pump Inhibitor Adverse Effects

The proposed risks of PPIs fall into 5 general categories. First, there has been concern that PPIs might increase the risk of developing some malignancies. Second, it has been proposed that PPIs increase the risk of developing a variety of infections. There are proposed PPI risks related to their effects on the absorption and metabolism of certain vitamins and minerals. PPI effects on the absorption and metabolism of certain drugs conceivably could have adverse consequences. Finally, there are an ever-increasing number of proposed miscellaneous adverse effects of PPIs.

Increased Risk of Malignancy

As discussed previously, gastrin can increase proliferation in ECL cells and the early finding that female rats treated lifelong with omeprazole developed hypergastrinemia, ECL cell hyperplasia, and gastric carcinoid (neuroendocrine) tumors delayed the release of omeprazole in the United States.[35] This concern about carcinoid tumors eventually was allayed by studies showing that animals other than female rats do not develop carcinoid tumors with PPI treatment, that PPI-induced hypergastrinemia in humans generally is mild, and that even severe hypergastrinemia rarely causes carcinoid tumors in human patients unless they have a genetic abnormality, such as multiple endocrine neoplasia 1.[36–38] Similarly, although gastrin increases proliferation in the colon, studies generally have not found an increase in colon cancer frequency among patients taking PPIs.[39,40]

For several reasons, it has been proposed that PPIs might be a risk factor for cancers in Barrett esophagus and in the stomach. Gastrin has been shown to increase proliferation in Barrett metaplasia, an effect that might promote the development of neoplasia.[32] Gastrin also increases ECL cell proliferation, and recent data suggest that some gastric adenocarcinomas might originate from ECL cells.[41] Acid suppression can enable colonization of the stomach by bacteria that deconjugate bile acids, and deconjugated bile acids that reflux into the esophagus can injure its mucosa and cause DNA damage.[42] Bacteria also can convert dietary nitrates into potentially carcinogenic N-nitroso compounds.[43] Finally, some studies have suggested that PPIs can accelerate the development of gastric atrophy in patients infected with *Helicobacter pylori*.[44] Although all these factors might be expected to promote carcinogenesis, few studies have linked PPI usage with the development of esophageal and gastric adenocarcinomas.[45–47] Furthermore, there are equally compelling reasons to suspect that PPI usage might protect against cancer in Barrett esophagus. Chronic inflammation is a risk factor for cancers in many organs, and PPIs heal the chronic esophageal inflammation of reflux esophagitis. Furthermore, acid can cause potentially carcinogenic DNA damage in Barrett esophagus,[48] and PPIs decrease esophageal acid exposure. Most, but not all studies on this issue suggest that PPIs protect against cancer in Barrett esophagus,[49,50] suggesting that PPI cancer-protective effects outweigh their potential to promote cancer in this condition.

Increased Risk of Infections

Gastric acid plays an important role in killing ingested microorganisms, and there are reports suggesting that acid suppression with PPIs might increase the risk of contracting enteric infections such as *Salmonella* and *Campylobacter*,[51] community-acquired pneumonias (perhaps due to colonization of the stomach with bacteria that might be refluxed and aspirated),[52] *Clostridium difficile* infections,[53] and spontaneous bacterial peritonitis in patients with cirrhosis (perhaps due to PPI-induced alterations in the gut microbiome that facilitate translocation of intestinal bacteria into ascetic fluid).[54] It is also conceivable that PPI anti-inflammatory effects contribute to the development of these infections.

Effects on Absorption and Metabolism of Vitamins and Minerals

PPIs can interfere with the absorption of vitamin B_{12}, iron and calcium. Acid-peptic activity is required to release dietary protein-bound cobalamin (vitamin B_{12}) so that it can bind to intrinsic factor and later be absorbed in the terminal ileum, and there are reports of patients on PPIs developing vitamin B_{12} deficiency.[55] Gastric acid facilitates oxidation of dietary ferric (Fe^{3+}) iron to ferrous iron (Fe^{2+}) that can be absorbed in the duodenum, and iron deficiency anemia has been reported in patients on PPI therapy.[56] Gastric acid also facilitates the absorption of calcium by inducing the ionization and solubilization of calcium salts, and it has been proposed that PPIs might increase the risk for osteoporosis and bone fractures by interfering with this process.[57,58] Hypomagnesemia also has been associated with PPI therapy, but the underlying mechanism is not clear.[59]

Effects on Absorption and Metabolism of Drugs

PPI-induced gastric acid suppression generally has little influence on drug absorption, with some notable exceptions. For example, ketoconazole may not be absorbed effectively without gastric acid and, conversely, elevated gastric pH levels facilitate the absorption of digoxin.[60] For patients requiring both PPI and antifungal therapy, clinicians should consider prescribing an agent other than ketoconazole, and for those treated concomitantly with PPIs and digoxin, clinicians should consider monitoring digoxin levels. PPIs are metabolized by the cytochrome P450 (CYP) system, and PPIs can affect the metabolism of other drugs metabolized by CYP enzymes.[61] Thus, PPIs can delay the clearance of warfarin, diazepam, and phenytoin, although clinically important drug interactions are uncommon.[62] PPIs also can delay the clearance of methotrexate, which is not metabolized importantly by CYP, possibly by interfering with hepatic and renal uptake of methotrexate via organic anion transporters.[63]

The potential for PPIs to reduce the antiplatelet action of clopidogrel has received considerable attention. Both PPIs and clopidogrel are metabolized by the CYP2C19 enzyme.[64] Unlike the PPIs, which are inactivated by CYP2C19, clopidogrel is a pro-drug that must be activated by CYP2C19 into a metabolite that inhibits platelet aggregation. For patients taking both drugs, therefore, the CYP2C19 used to inactivate the PPI might not be available to activate the clopidogrel, thus decreasing its antiplatelet effect. This interaction can be demonstrated using blood tests of platelet function in patients taking both PPIs and clopidogrel, but the clinical importance of the interaction remains disputed.[65] In 2009, a large, retrospective cohort study of patients who had been hospitalized for acute coronary syndrome found that the frequency of death or recurrent acute coronary syndrome was significantly higher in those who took clopidogrel concomitantly with a PPI.[66] Most subsequent observational studies on the safety of PPIs used with dual antiplatelet therapy (generally aspirin and clopidogrel) also have found more ischemic events in patients taking clopidogrel with PPIs.[67] Based on such data, the US Food and Drug Administration has issued warnings to avoid using omeprazole or esomeprazole with clopidogrel. Several randomized controlled trials, however, have found no significant differences in cardiovascular outcomes for patients taking clopidogrel with or without omeprazole.[67] Unfortunately, none of those trials was sufficiently powered to exclude a small but potentially important difference in the frequency of cardiovascular events due to use of PPIs.

Miscellaneous Adverse Effects

Reports of miscellaneous, unanticipated adverse effects of PPIs have increased dramatically in frequency over the past several years. These include diverse conditions, such as myocardial infarction, stroke, acute and chronic kidney disease, microscopic colitis, EoE, celiac diseases, dementia, and even early death.

As described previously, the increased frequency of cardiovascular events observed in patients taking clopidogrel together with PPIs initially was explained by the drugs competing for metabolism by CYP2C19. A large study of patients with acute coronary syndrome who were treated with ticagrelor, an antiplatelet agent that is not metabolized by CYP2C19, also found an increased frequency of adverse cardiovascular events in patients concomitantly taking PPIs.[68] Other studies have described increased adverse cardiovascular events even in GERD patients who take PPIs, also suggesting that PPIs might have cardiovascular effects independent of their effects on clopidogrel activation.[69] One proposed explanation involves complicated PPI effects that result in decreased production of nitric oxide and altered vascular homeostasis.[70]

Acute interstitial nephritis is often an idiosyncratic drug hypersensitivity reaction, and more than 250 drugs, including the PPIs, have been implicated as causative agents.[71] Acute interstitial nephritis can cause severe kidney injury that progresses to chronic kidney disease. PPI use has been associated with chronic kidney disease, although it is not clear that progression of acute interstitial nephritis is the underlying mechanism in all cases.[72,73]

It has been proposed that PPIs might contribute to the development of EoE through their effects on peptic digestion and on gastric permeability.[74] PPIs raise gastric pH to levels at which pepsin is not active (ie, pH >4), and, consequently, ingested peptides that are not degraded by pepsin in the stomach might evoke an allergic response when they reach the small intestine. Furthermore, PPIs increase gastric mucosal permeability, thereby facilitating the uptake of undegraded peptide allergens and their exposure to immune cells. The aforementioned PPI effects on the gut microbiome also might predispose to EoE development. Similar mechanisms that might alter the degradation and immunogenicity of dietary gluten have been proposed to explain the association of celiac disease with PPI usage.[75] Conceivably, such mechanisms also might underlie the proposed association of PPIs with microscopic colitis.[76] A role for PPIs in the pathogenesis of EoE might seem paradoxic because PPIs are used to treat EoE. The mechanisms proposed to explain the beneficial effects of PPIs in EoE (ie, blocking T_H2 cytokine-stimulated production of eotaxin-3), however, are entirely different than those proposed to explain their role in EoE pathogenesis.

The accumulation of β-amyloid peptide in the brain is believed to play a major pathogenetic role in Alzheimer disease. Normally, microglia in the brain engulf β-amyloid peptide deposits and degrade them in lysosomes that are acidified by vacuolar proton pumps (V-ATPases), which are susceptible to inhibition by PPIs. It has been proposed that PPIs might be a risk factor for dementia because they hamper the degradation of β-amyloid peptide by preventing acidification of microglial lysosomes.[77]

Finally, PPI use has been associated with increased risk of all-cause mortality.[78] It is not clear which, if any, of these mechanisms might contribute to this putative excess risk of death.

PROBLEMS WITH STUDIES IDENTIFYING PROTON PUMP INHIBITOR RISKS

The putative risks of PPIs, described previously, were identified primarily as weak associations found in observational studies, and there are contradictory reports regarding the validity of each of those putative risks. Observational studies are notoriously unreliable for identifying important cause-and-effect relationships. In a report entitled, "False Alarms and Pseudo-Epidemics: The Limitations of Observational Epidemiology," Grimes and Schulz point out that "most reported associations in observational clinical research are false, and the minority of associations that are true are often exaggerated."[79] They go on to note, "This issue is especially problematic for weak associations…[which] are more likely to be attributable to bias than to causal association…In general, unless relative risks in cohort studies exceed 2 to 3, or odds ratios in case-control studies exceed 3 or 4, associations in observational research findings should not be considered credible." Most of the putative PPI risks, discussed previously, were identified in studies with relative risks and odds ratios considerably below those limits.

Unfortunately, even strong associations found in observational studies cannot establish cause and effect because of the substantial biases that often confound those studies. For example, some observational studies have identified a strong association (odds ratios >4) between PPI usage and the development of esophageal adenocarcinoma.[80] One possible conclusion for this observation is that PPIs are a risk factor for esophageal cancer. GERD, however, is a well-established, strong risk factor for esophageal adenocarcinoma, and PPIs are commonly prescribed to treat GERD. Consequently, it seems more likely that the indication for the PPI prescription (ie, GERD) is the important cancer risk factor, not the PPIs used to treat GERD. This is an example of confounding by indication, a bias that often is difficult to exclude in observational studies on putative PPI side effects.

Observational studies also have found strong associations between PPIs and community-acquired pneumonias, and 1 possible conclusion is that PPIs are a risk factor for those pneumonias. Cough and chest discomfort, however, are early symptoms of pneumonia, and physicians often prescribe PPIs to treat cough and chest discomfort. Consequently, in observational studies that identified an association between PPI use and community-acquired pneumonia, it is possible that the PPIs did not cause the infection but were prescribed for the early symptoms of pneumonia. This is an example of protopathic bias, which may well explain the association of PPIs and community-acquired pneumonia. A nested case-control study on this issue that used the UK General Practice Research Database found that the odds ratio for this association decreased as the length of time between the PPI prescription and the occurrence of pneumonia increased.[81] There was a strong association (adjusted odds ratio 6.53; CI, 3.95–10.80) when the PPIs were started within 2 days of the diagnosis of pneumonia, but there was no significant association between long-term PPI usage and pneumonia (adjusted odds ratio 1.02; CI, 0.97–1,08). These findings strongly suggest protopathic bias, with PPIs not playing a pathogenetic role but merely prescribed for the early symptoms of a pneumonia already present.

Although associations found in observational studies can never establish cause-and-effect relationships, in 1965, Sir Austin Hill[82] proposed a list of 9 considerations that can strengthen the case for cause and effect. These include

1. Strength of the association
2. Consistency (ie, the findings are reproducible)
3. Specificity (ie, there are few or no alternative factors to explain the association)
4. Temporality (ie, the risk factor precedes the disorder)
5. Biological gradient (ie, there is a dose and duration response)
6. Biological plausibility (ie, there is a reasonable mechanism)
7. Coherence (ie, different types of evidence agree)
8. Experiment (ie, there are experimental data that support the association)
9. Analogy (ie, there is an association between the disorder and a similar risk factor)

A recent review by Vaezi and colleagues[83] found that none of the associations between PPI use and their putative serious adverse effects fulfilled all of the Hill criteria, and most fulfilled only 1 or 2 of the 9.

SUMMARY

Observational studies on PPI risks can establish associations but cannot establish cause-and-effect relationships, and observational studies are highly susceptible to bias. The proposed risks of PPIs have been identified largely as weak associations in flawed observational studies, and the putative underlying mechanisms often are dubious. As weak as the evidence might be, however, the risks generally cannot be dismissed out of hand. With so much smoke, there could well be some real fires. Weak association does not strongly support causality, but it does not exclude it either. Nor does weak association equate to a lack of clinical importance. Even a small increase in the risk of a catastrophic event like myocardial infarction or stroke is important and, unfortunately, the uncertainty about PPI risks is unlikely to be resolved any time in the near future.

The best way to avoid drug side effects is to not prescribe a drug unless there is a clear indication and then to use it in the recommended dosage. For the conditions listed in **Box 1**, there is general consensus that the benefits of PPIs clearly outweigh their potential risks. As discussed previously, however, PPIs often are used inappropriately and often are prescribed in higher-than-recommended dosages. Before prescribing PPIs, physicians should carefully consider whether there is a valid indication (see **Box 1**) and, if there is, to confirm the appropriate dosing for the condition. For patients already taking PPIs, the physician should carefully review the medical record and determine whether continuation of PPI therapy is appropriate. Such a review often reveals that PPIs should be discontinued.

REFERENCES

1. Naunton M, Peterson GM, Deeks LS, et al. We have had a gutful: the need for deprescribing proton pump inhibitors. J Clin Pharm Ther 2018;43:65–72.
2. Kantor ED, Rehm CD, Haas JS, et al. Trends in prescription drug use among adults in the United States from 1999-2012. JAMA 2015;314:1818–31.
3. Hersey SJ, Sachs G. Gastric acid secretion. Physiol Rev 1995;75:155–89.
4. Shin JM, Sachs G. Pharmacology of proton pump inhibitors. Curr Gastroenterol Rep 2008;10:528–34.
5. Peghini PL, Katz PO, Castell DO. Ranitidine controls nocturnal gastric acid breakthrough on omeprazole: a controlled study in normal subjects. Gastroenterology 1998;115:1335–9.
6. Ours TM, Fackler WK, Richter JE, et al. Nocturnal acid breakthrough: clinical significance and correlation with esophageal acid exposure. Am J Gastroenterol 2003;98:545–50.
7. Hershcovici T, Jha LK, Fass R. Dexlansoprazole MR: a review. Ann Med 2011;43: 366–74.
8. Katz PO, Koch FK, Ballard ED, et al. Comparison of the effects of immediate-release omeprazole oral suspension, delayed-release lansoprazole capsules and delayed-release esomeprazole capsules on nocturnal gastric acidity after bedtime dosing in patients with night-time GERD symptoms. Aliment Pharmacol Ther 2007;25:197–205.
9. Katz PO. Review article: putting immediate-release proton-pump inhibitors into clinical practice–improving nocturnal acid control and avoiding the possible complications of excessive acid exposure. Aliment Pharmacol Ther 2005;22(Suppl 3): 31–8.
10. Kedika RR, Souza RF, Spechler SJ. Potential anti-inflammatory effects of the proton pump inhibitors: a review and discussion of the clinical implications. Dig Dis Sci 2009;54:2312–7.
11. Biswas K, Bandyopadhyay U, Chattopadhyay I, et al. A novel antioxidant and antiapoptotic role of omeprazole to block gastric ulcer through scavenging of hydroxyl radical. J Biol Chem 2003;278:10993–1001.
12. Pastoris O, Verri M, Boschi F, et al. Effects of esomeprazole on glutathione levels and mitochondrial oxidative phosphorylation in the gastric mucosa of rats treated with indomethacin. Naunyn Schmiedebergs Arch Pharmacol 2008;378:421–9.
13. Becker JC, Grosser N, Waltke C, et al. Beyond gastric acid reduction: proton pump inhibitors induce heme oxygenase-1 in gastric and endothelial cells. Biochem Biophys Res Commun 2006;345:1014–21.
14. Suzuki M, Mori M, Miura S, et al. Omeprazole attenuates oxygen-derived free radical production from human neutrophils. Free Radic Biol Med 1996;21:727–31.
15. Zedtwitz-Liebenstein K, Wenisch C, Patruta S, et al. Omeprazole treatment diminishes intra- and extracellular neutrophil reactive oxygen production and bactericidal activity. Crit Care Med 2002;30:1118–22.
16. Wandall JH. Effects of omeprazole on neutrophil chemotaxis, super oxide production, degranulation, and translocation of cytochrome b-245. Gut 1992;33: 617–21.
17. Handa O, Yoshida N, Fujita N, et al. Molecular mechanisms involved in anti-inflammatory effects of proton pump inhibitors. Inflamm Res 2006;55:476–80.
18. Suzuki M, Nakamura M, Mori M, et al. Lansoprazole inhibits oxygen-derived free radical production from neutrophils activated by Helicobacter pylori. J Clin Gastroenterol 1995;20(Suppl 2):S93–6.

19. Martins de Oliveira R, Antunes E, Pedrazzoli J Jr, et al. The inhibitory effects of H+ K+ ATPase inhibitors on human neutrophils in vitro: restoration by a K+ iono-phore. Inflamm Res 2007;56:105–11.

20. Barthel SR, Annis DS, Mosher DF, et al. Differential engagement of modules 1 and 4 of vascular cell adhesion molecule-1 (CD106) by integrins alpha4beta1 (CD49d/29) and alphaMbeta2 (CD11b/18) of eosinophils. J Biol Chem 2006; 281:32175–87.

21. Sasaki T, Yamaya M, Yasuda H, et al. The proton pump inhibitor lansoprazole in-hibits rhinovirus infection in cultured human tracheal epithelial cells. Eur J Phar-macol 2005;509(2–3):201–10.

22. Furuta GT, Liacouras CA, Collins MH, et al, First International Gastrointestinal Eosinophil Research Symposium (FIGERS) Subcommittees. Eosinophilic esoph-agitis in children and adults: a systematic review and consensus recommenda-tions for diagnosis and treatment. Gastroenterology 2007;133:1342–63.

23. Cheng E, Zhang X, Huo X, et al. Omeprazole blocks eotaxin-3 expression by oe-sophageal squamous cells from patients with eosinophilic oesophagitis and GORD. Gut 2013;62:824–32.

24. Scarpignato C, Gatta L, Zullo A, et al, SIF-AIGO-FIMMG Group, Italian Society of Pharmacology, the Italian Association of Hospital Gastroenterologists, and the Italian Federation of General Practitioners. Effective and safe proton pump inhib-itor therapy in acid-related diseases – a position paper addressing benefits and potential harms of acid suppression. BMC Med 2016;14:179.

25. Dunbar KB, Agoston AT, Odze RD, et al. Association of acute gastroesophageal reflux disease with esophageal histologic changes. JAMA 2016;315:2104–12.

26. Lanza FL, Chan FK, Quigley EM. Practice Parameters Committee of the American College of Gastroenterology. Guidelines for prevention of NSAID-related ulcer complications. Am J Gastroenterol 2009;104(3):728–38.

27. Chia CT, Lim WP, Vu CK. Inappropriate use of proton pump inhibitors in a local setting. Singapore Med J 2014;55:363–6.

28. Molloy D, Molloy A, O'Loughlin C, et al. Inappropriate use of proton pump inhib-itors. Ir J Med Sci 2010;179:73–5.

29. Naito Y, Kashiwagi K, Takagi T, et al. Intestinal dysbiosis secondary to proton-pump inhibitor use. Digestion 2018;97:195–204.

30. Lundell L, Vieth M, Gibson F, et al. Systematic review: the effects of long-term pro-ton pump inhibitor use on serum gastrin levels and gastric histology. Aliment Pharmacol Ther 2015;42:649–63.

31. Dockray GJ, Varro A, Dimaline R, et al. The gastrins: their production and biolog-ical activities. Annu Rev Physiol 2001;63:119–39.

32. Haigh CR, Attwood SE, Thompson DG, et al. Gastrin induces proliferation in Bar-rett's metaplasia through activation of the CCK2 receptor. Gastroenterology 2003; 124:615–25.

33. Waldum HL, Arnestad JS, Brenna E, et al. Marked increase in gastric acid secre-tory capacity after omeprazole treatment. Gut 1996;39:649–53.

34. Fossmark R, Johnsen G, Johanessen E, et al. Rebound acid hypersecretion after long-term inhibition of gastric acid secretion. Aliment Pharmacol Ther 2005;21: 149–54.

35. Havu N. Enterochromaffin-like cell carcinoids of gastric mucosa in rats after life-long inhibition of gastric secretion. Digestion 1986;35(Suppl 1):42–55.

36. Freston JW. Clinical significance of hypergastrinaemia: relevance to gastrin moni-toring during omeprazole therapy. Digestion 1992;51(Suppl 1):102–14.

37. Solcia E, Capella C, Fiocca R, et al. Gastric argyrophil carcinoidosis in patients with Zollinger-Ellison syndrome due to type 1 multiple endocrine neoplasia. A newly recognized association. Am J Surg Pathol 1990;4:503–13.
38. Laine L, Ahnen D, McClain C, et al. Review article: potential gastrointestinal effects of long-term acid suppression with proton pump inhibitors. Aliment Pharmacol Ther 2000;14:651–8.
39. Singh M, Dhindsa G, Friedland S, et al. Long-term use of proton pump inhibitors does not affect the frequency, growth, or histologic characteristics of colon adenomas. Aliment Pharmacol Ther 2007;26:1051–61.
40. Ahn JS, Park SM, Eom CS, et al. Use of proton pump inhibitor and risk of colorectal cancer: a meta-analysis of observational studies. Korean J Fam Med 2012;33:272–9.
41. Waldum HL, Sørdal Ø, Fossmark R. Proton pump inhibitors (PPIs) may cause gastric cancer - clinical consequences. Scand J Gastroenterol 2018;53(6): 639–42.
42. Theisen J, Nehra D, Citron D, et al. Suppression of gastric acid secretion in patients with gastroesophageal reflux disease results in gastric bacterial overgrowth and deconjugation of bile acids. J Gastrointest Surg 2000;4:50–4.
43. Calmels S, Béréziat JC, Ohshima H, et al. Bacterial formation of N-nitroso compounds from administered precursors in the rat stomach after omeprazole-induced achlorhydria. Carcinogenesis 1991;12:435–9.
44. Kuipers EJ, Lee A, Klinkenberg-Knol EC, et al. Review article: the development of atrophic gastritis–Helicobacter pylori and the effects of acid suppressive therapy. Aliment Pharmacol Ther 1995;9:331–40.
45. Cheung KS, Chan EW, Wong AYS, et al. Long-term proton pump inhibitors and risk of gastric cancer development after treatment for Helicobacter pylori: a population-based study. Gut 2018;67:28–35.
46. Brusselaers N, Wahlin K, Engstrand L, et al. Maintenance therapy with proton pump inhibitors and risk of gastric cancer: a nationwide population-based cohort study in Sweden. BMJ Open 2017;7:e017739.
47. Brusselaers N, Engstrand L, Lagergren J. Maintenance proton pump inhibition therapy and risk of oesophageal cancer. Cancer Epidemiol 2018;53:172–7.
48. Zhang HY, Hormi-Carver K, Zhang X, et al. In benign Barrett's epithelial cells, acid exposure generates reactive oxygen species that cause DNA double strand breaks. Cancer Res 2009;69:9083–9.
49. Singh S, Garg SK, Singh PP, et al. Acid-suppressive medications and risk of oesophageal adenocarcinoma in patients with Barrett's oesophagus: a systematic review and meta-analysis. Gut 2014;63:1229–37.
50. Hu Q, Sun TT, Hong J, et al. Proton pump inhibitors do not reduce the risk of esophageal adenocarcinoma in patients with Barrett's esophagus: a systematic review and meta-analysis. PLoS One 2017;12(1):e0169691.
51. Bavishi C, Dupont HL. Systematic review: the use of proton pump inhibitors and increased susceptibility to enteric infection. Aliment Pharmacol Ther 2011;34: 1269–81.
52. Lambert AA, Lam JO, Paik JJ, et al. Risk of community-acquired pneumonia with outpatient proton-pump inhibitor therapy: a systematic review and meta-analysis. PLoS One 2015;10:e0128004.
53. Kwok CS, Arthur AK, Anibueze CI, et al. Risk of Clostridium difficile infection with acid suppressing drugs and antibiotics: meta-analysis. Am J Gastroenterol 2012; 107:1011–9.

54. Deshpande A, Pasupuleti V, Thota P, et al. Acid-suppressive therapy is associated with spontaneous bacterial peritonitis in cirrhotic patients: a meta-analysis. J Gastroenterol Hepatol 2013;28:235–42.

55. Lam JR, Schneider JL, Zhao W, et al. Proton pump inhibitor and histamine 2 receptor antagonist use and vitamin B12 deficiency. JAMA 2013;310:2435–42.

56. Sarzynski E, Puttarajappa C, Xie Y, et al. Association between proton pump inhibitor use and anemia: a retrospective cohort study. Dig Dis Sci 2011;56:2349–53.

57. Andersen BN, Johansen PB, Abrahamsen B. Proton pump inhibitors and osteoporosis. Curr Opin Rheumatol 2016;28:420–5.

58. Ngamruengphong S, Leontiadis GI, Radhi S, et al. Proton pump inhibitors and risk of fracture: a systematic review and meta-analysis of observational studies. Am J Gastroenterol 2011;106:1209–18.

59. William JH, Danziger J. Proton-pump inhibitor-induced hypomagnesemia: current research and proposed mechanisms. World J Nephrol 2016;5:152–7.

60. Lew EA. Review article: pharmacokinetic concerns in the selection of anti-ulcer therapy. Aliment Pharmacol Ther 1999;13(suppl 5):11–6.

61. VandenBranden M, Ring BJ, Binkley SN, et al. Interaction of human liver cytochromes P450 in vitro with LY307640, a gastric proton pump inhibitor. Pharmacogenetics 1996;6:81–91.

62. Humphries TJ, Merritt GJ. Review article: drug interactions with agents used to treat acid-related diseases. Aliment Pharmacol Ther 1999;13(suppl 3):18–26.

63. Bezabeh S, Mackey AC, Kluetz P, et al. Accumulating evidence for a drug-drug interaction between methotrexate and proton pump inhibitors. Oncologist 2012; 17:550–4.

64. Gilard M, Arnaud B, Le Gal G, et al. Influence of omeprazole on the antiplatelet action of clopidogrel associated to aspirin. J Thromb Haemost 2006;4:2508–9.

65. Gilard M, Arnaud B, Cornily JC, et al. Influence of omeprazole on the antiplatelet action of clopidogrel associated with aspirin: the randomized, double-blind OCLA (Omeprazole CLopidogrel Aspirin) study. J Am Coll Cardiol 2008;51: 256–60.

66. Ho PM, Maddox TM, Wang L, et al. Risk of adverse outcomes associated with concomitant use of clopidogrel and proton pump inhibitors following acute coronary syndrome. JAMA 2009;301:937–44.

67. Melloni C, Washam JB, Jones WS, et al. Conflicting results between randomized trials and observational studies on the impact of proton pump inhibitors on cardiovascular events when coadministered with dual antiplatelet therapy: systematic review. Circ Cardiovasc Qual Outcomes 2015;8:47–55.

68. Goodman SG, Clare R, Pieper KS, et al, Platelet Inhibition and Patient Outcomes Trial Investigators. Association of proton pump inhibitor use on cardiovascular outcomes with clopidogrel and ticagrelor: insights from the platelet inhibition and patient outcomes trial. Circulation 2012;125:978–86.

69. Sun S, Cui Z, Zhou M, et al. Proton pump inhibitor monotherapy and the risk of cardiovascular events in patients with gastro-esophageal reflux disease: a meta-analysis. Neurogastroenterol Motil 2017;29(2).

70. Ghebremariam YT, LePendu P, Lee JC, et al. Unexpected effect of proton pump inhibitors: elevation of the cardiovascular risk factor asymmetric dimethylarginine. Circulation 2013;128:845–53.

71. Raghavan R, Shawar S. Mechanisms of drug-induced interstitial nephritis. Adv Chronic Kidney Dis 2017;24:64–71.

72. Yang Y, George KC, Shang WF, et al. Proton pump inhibitors use, and risk of acute kidney injury: a meta-analysis of observational studies. Drug Des Devel Ther 2017;11:1291–9.
73. Nochaiwong S, Ruengorn C, Awiphan R, et al. The association between proton pump inhibitor use and the risk of adverse kidney outcomes: a systematic review and meta-analysis. Nephrol Dial Transplant 2018;33:331–42.
74. Merwat SN, Spechler SJ. Might the use of acid suppressive medications predispose to the development of eosinophilic esophagitis? Am J Gastroenterol 2009; 104:1897–902.
75. Lebwohl B, Spechler SJ, Wang TC, et al. Use of proton pump inhibitors and subsequent risk of celiac disease. Dig Liver Dis 2014;46:36–40.
76. Law EH, Badowski M, Hung YT, et al. Association between proton pump inhibitors and microscopic colitis. Ann Pharmacother 2017;51:253–63.
77. Fallahzadeh MK, Borhani Haghighi A, Namazi MR. Proton pump inhibitors: predisposers to Alzheimer disease? J Clin Pharm Ther 2010;35:125–6.
78. Xie Y, Bowe B, Li T, et al. Risk of death among users of Proton Pump Inhibitors: a longitudinal observational cohort study of United States veterans. BMJ Open 2017;7(6):e015735.
79. Grimes DA, Schulz KF. False alarms and pseudo-epidemics: the limitations of observational epidemiology. Obstet Gynecol 2012;120:920–7.
80. García Rodríguez LA, Lagergren J, Lindblad M. Gastric acid suppression and risk of oesophageal and gastric adenocarcinoma: a nested case control study in the UK. Gut 2006;55:1538–44.
81. Sarkar M, Hennessy S, Yang YX. Proton-pump inhibitor use and the risk for community-acquired pneumonia. Ann Intern Med 2008;149:391–8.
82. Hill AB. The environment and disease: association or causation? 1965. J R Soc Med 2015;108:32–7.
83. Vaezi MF, Yang YX, Howden CW. Complications of proton pump inhibitor therapy. Gastroenterology 2017;153:35–48.

Proton Pump Inhibitor– Refractory Gastroesophageal Reflux Disease

Rena Yadlapati, MD, MSHS*, Kelli DeLay, MD

KEYWORDS

- PPI-refractory • Antireflux surgery • Fundoplication
- Magnetic sphincter augmentation • Gastroesophageal reflux disease (GERD)

KEY POINTS

- Proton pump inhibitor (PPI)-refractory gastroesophageal reflux disease (GERD) occurs when troublesome symptoms and elevated acid exposure and/or reflux burden persist despite an optimized PPI trial.
- PPI-refractory GERD arises from dysfunction of physiologic lines of defense (eg, antireflux barrier, reflux clearance, epithelial tissue resistance) and propagation of reflux mechanisms (eg, transient lower esophageal sphincter relaxations, hernia re-reflux, hypotensive lower esophageal sphincter [LES]).
- Pharmacologic options for PPI-refractory GERD include switching to a less cytochrome P2C19–dependent PPI, adding histamine-2 receptor antagonists at night, using alginate-based antacids, and trialing gamma-aminobutyric acid agonists.
- Surgical options for PPI-refractory GERD include laparoscopic fundoplication, magnetic sphincter augmentation, and Roux-en-Y gastric bypass, particularly in the setting of morbid obesity.
- Transoral incisionless fundoplication and radiofrequency energy delivery to the LES are endoluminal interventional options for PPI-refractory GERD.

INTRODUCTION

Gastroesophageal reflux disease (GERD) is among the most common conditions seen in ambulatory clinics and its disease burden continues to increase, with most recent studies reporting an 18% to 28% prevalence of GERD among North Americans.[1,2]

Disclosures: R. Yadlapati is supported by NIH R01 DK092217 and the American College of Gastroenterology 2018 Junior Faculty Development Award. R. Yadlapati consults for Ironwood Pharmaceuticals, Medtronic, and Diversatek Healthcare.
Division of Gastroenterology and Hepatology, University of Colorado Anschutz Medical Campus, 12631 East 17th Avenue B158, Aurora, CO 80045, USA
* Corresponding author.
E-mail address: Rena.Yadlapati@UCDenver.edu

Med Clin N Am 103 (2019) 15–27
https://doi.org/10.1016/j.mcna.2018.08.002
0025-7125/19/Published by Elsevier Inc.

medical.theclinics.com

Proton pump inhibitor (PPI) therapy is the mainstay pharmacologic management for GERD, although up to 40% of patients with suspected GERD derive inadequate symptom relief with PPI.[3] Although patients with PPI nonresponse may not have true GERD to begin with, a subset of PPI nonresponders will have PPI-refractory GERD. The management strategies for refractory GERD expand beyond PPIs to include other pharmacologic or invasive interventions. Because mechanisms of PPI-refractory GERD are varied, the choice of management strategy should be personalized to the patient's needs and mechanistic dysfunction. This article reviews the definition, mechanisms, and management options for PPI-refractory GERD.

DEFINITION OF PROTON PUMP INHIBITOR–REFRACTORY GASTROESOPHAGEAL REFLUX DISEASE

PPI-refractory GERD is defined as the presence of persistent troublesome GERD symptoms and objective evidence of GERD despite optimized PPI therapy (**Fig. 1**). Generally, an optimized PPI trial consists of double-dose PPI therapy over at least 8 weeks.[4] Data supporting the optimal duration and dose of a PPI trial mostly derive from studies assessing healing in erosive esophagitis, which demonstrated higher rates of endoscopic healing of erosive esophagitis and heartburn symptom resolution with double-dose PPI compared with single-dose PPI,[5] and lower symptom relapse following 8 weeks of PPI therapy compared with 4 weeks of therapy.[6] Currently, the US Food and Drug Administration (FDA) recommends single-dose PPI use over 4 to 8 weeks for GERD.[7] Professional societies, such as the American College of Gastroenterology and the American Gastroenterological Association, recommend escalating to double-dose PPI if erosive esophagitis persists or symptoms are only partially controlled on single-dose PPI.[8,9]

Partial PPI response, according to the Montreal Consensus, is the presence of mild heartburn and/or regurgitation on 3 or more days per week despite at least 4 weeks of

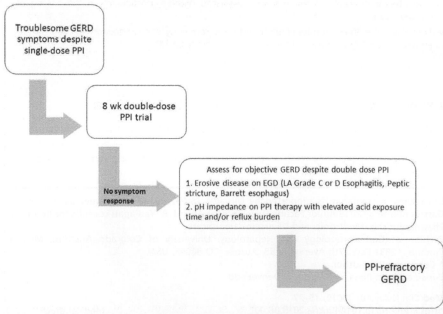

Fig. 1. Arriving at a diagnosis of PPI-refractory GERD. EGD, Esophagogastroduodenoscopy.

PPI.[10] When assessing for symptom response it is essential to ensure correct medication administration and that PPIs are being taken 30 to 60 minutes before a meal because up to 54% of patients take PPIs incorrectly.[11,12] Furthermore, at the onset of treatment, providers should review treatment expectations and assist with goal-setting. An aligned goal should be to reduce symptoms to a tolerable level and optimize quality of life, with the shared understanding that complete resolution is rarely achieved.[13]

Objective Diagnosis of Proton Pump Inhibitor–Refractory Gastroesophageal Reflux Disease

In the setting of persistent troublesome symptoms despite an appropriate PPI trial, the next step is to evaluate for objective evidence of GERD. Esophageal pH monitoring is the gold standard, and the choice of testing modality depends on the posttest likelihood of GERD. If objective GERD has not been previously diagnosed and/or there is a low suspicion of pathologic GERD, initial testing should be performed off PPI therapy with either wireless or catheter-based pH systems to evaluate for baseline GERD.[14] Not infrequently, pH testing in these scenarios is negative for GERD and helps to guide the evaluation and management away from GERD. However, in patients previously diagnosed with pathologic GERD (eg, Los Angeles Grade C or D esophagitis, peptic stricture, Barrett esophagus, or pathologic acid exposure off PPI on esophageal pH monitoring) the diagnostic evaluation begins with esophageal pH-impedance monitoring on PPI therapy to assess not only for PPI-refractory acid exposure but also excessive burden of nonacidic or weakly acidic contents.[14] According to the GERD Consensus Group, esophageal acid exposure time greater than 6% on PPI is consistent with PPI-refractory GERD. When acid exposure time is borderline (4%–6%), the group recommends consideration of further complimentary metrics (**Fig. 2**).

MECHANISMS OF PROTON PUMP INHIBITOR–REFRACTORY GASTROESOPHAGEAL REFLUX DISEASE

Pathologic GERD typically requires compromise to 1 or more protective systems that exist to prevent gastroesophageal reflux, as well as an enhanced reflux physiology (**Table 1**).

Antireflux Barrier

The antireflux barrier is a high-pressure zone made up of the lower esophageal sphincter (LES) attached to the crural diaphragm via the phrenoesophageal ligament

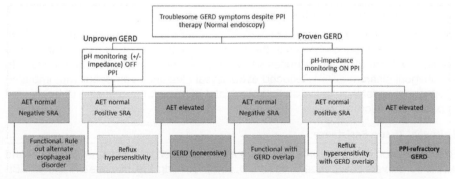

Fig. 2. Role of pH testing to identify causes of PPI nonresponse. AET, Acid Exposure Time; SRA, Symptom-Reflux Association.

Table 1
Diagnostic testing and management options based on pathophysiologic mechanism of proton pump inhibitor–refractory gastroesophageal reflux disease

Pathophysiologic Mechanism	Presenting Symptoms	Diagnostic Testing	Potential Treatment Options
Increased TLESR	Regurgitation, heartburn, chest pain	Postprandial high-resolution esophageal manometry	GABA agonist
Hiatal hernia	Regurgitation, heartburn, chest pain	Barium esophagram; upper GI endoscopy; high-resolution esophageal manometry	Hernia repair
Hypotensive LES	Regurgitation, heartburn, chest pain	High-resolution esophageal manometry	Surgical or endoluminal restoration
Reduced esophageal contractility	Dysphagia	High-resolution esophageal manometry	Limited options Consider muscarinic receptor agonist
Increased mucosal permeability	Heartburn	Mucosal impedance testing (investigational); pH impedance testing	—
Persistent esophageal acid exposure on double-dose PPI	Heartburn, chest pain	pH impedance testing on PPI	H2RA Consider switching to a CYP-independent PPI
Delayed gastric emptying	Regurgitation, heartburn, chest pain	Gastric emptying study; upper GI series with small bowel follow-through	Roux-en-Y gastric bypass

Abbreviations: CYP, cytochrome P; GABA, gamma-aminobutyric acid; GI, gastrointestinal; H2RA, histamine-2 receptor antagonist; LES, lower esophageal sphincter; TLESR, transient lower esophageal sphincter relaxation.

and functions to prevent gastroesophageal reflux. Reduced integrity of the antireflux barrier, either by way of a hypotonic resting LES and/or axial displacement of the LES and crural diaphragm (hiatal hernia), can lead to increased reflux burden and acid exposure (**Fig. 3**).[15,16]

Reduced Esophageal Clearance

Delays in esophageal acid and bolus clearance are also associated with pathologic acid reflux.[17] Primary peristalsis is the principal mechanism of reflux clearance.[18] In addition, volume distention induces secondary peristalsis and salivation assists with esophageal clearance.[19,20] Reduced esophageal clearance can occur with impaired esophageal peristalsis, in the setting of a hiatal hernia with re-refluxing of bolus, and impaired salivation.[21]

Epithelial Tissue Resistance

Barrier function of the esophageal mucosa is maintained by cell-to-cell junctions and works to prevent toxic substances from compromising the mucosal integrity.[22] Biopsies in patients with erosive and nonerosive reflux disease show evidence of microscopic esophagitis: necrosis, erosions, eosinophilic or neutrophilic infiltrate, basal cell

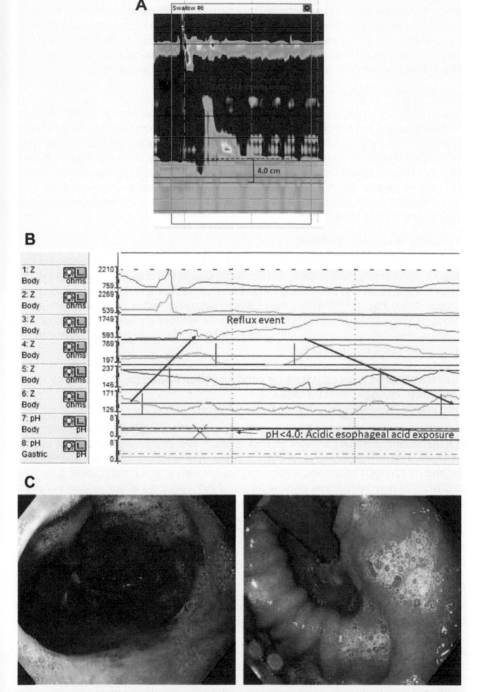

Fig. 3. A patient with troublesome regurgitation and heartburn despite optimized PPI therapy for 8 weeks and a previously positive wireless pH study performed off PPI previously was noted on evaluation to have a 4.0 cm hiatal hernia and pathologic gastroesophageal reflux.

hyperplasia, elongation of papillae, or dilation of intercellular spaces.[23] Therefore, reduced mucosal integrity is a potential mechanism of PPI-refractory GERD. Mucosal impedance is an emerging field of study to examine electrical conductivity and mucosal integrity of the esophagus. A lower baseline mucosal impedance is associated with increased acid exposure and dilated intracellular spaces, and seems to differentiate patients with objective GERD from other disease states.[24,25]

Delayed Gastric Emptying

Slowed gastric emptying may also contribute to PPI-refractory GERD through increased gastric distension and initiation of reflux events via transient LES relaxations (TLESRs).[26] In 1 study, use of a prokinetic agent that accelerates gastric emptying before pH-impedance and manometry testing significantly reduced acid exposure time and acid clearance time.[27] However, in the absence of delayed gastric emptying, the data generally do not demonstrate reliable symptom improvement in PPI-refractory GERD with adjunctive use of promotility agents (ie, metoclopramide, prucalopride, and domperidone).[28,29]

Physiologic Mechanisms of Reflux

TLESRs, prolonged relaxations in the LES associated with inhibition of the crural diaphragm that occur in response to gastric distention in the absence of a swallow, are the primary mechanism of initiating reflux in the context of an intact esophagogastric junction (EGJ) (**Fig. 4**).[29–32] When the LES is hypotensive, reflux can occur with an increase in intragastric pressure (strain-induced) or without an increase in intragastric pressure (free-reflux). Furthermore, gastric contents and esophageal bolus can re-reflux when hiatal hernia is present.

PHARMACOLOGIC MANAGEMENT OF PROTON PUMP INHIBITOR–REFRACTORY GASTROESOPHAGEAL REFLUX DISEASE
Cytochrome P–Independent Proton Pump Inhibitors

The mainstay of treatment of GERD is PPIs. Among different PPIs, there are variations in drug metabolism that can alter plasma levels.[33] Genetic polymorphisms of the cytochrome P (CYP) isoenzyme CYP2C19 in the liver affect drug levels of PPIs that depend on CYP2C19 for metabolism.[34] A patient with a rapid metabolizer genotype of CYP2C19 may have lower plasma levels of PPI, reducing effective acid suppression.[35] Use of specific PPIs that do not rely exclusively on CYP2C19 metabolism (ie, rabeprazole and esomeprazole) in rapid metabolizers can increase acid suppression, improve symptom response, and improve rates of healing and remission of erosive esophagitis.[32,36] Therefore, switching therapy from CYP-dependent PPIs to more CYP-independent PPIs in partial PPI responders may be a reasonable first step.[32,37]

Histamine-2 Receptor Antagonists

Histamine-2 receptor antagonists (H2RAs) can be used to help reduce nighttime heartburn in conjunction with double-dose PPI.[32,38] Although there is controversy

The patient underwent a hernia repair and magnetic sphincter augmentation. (A) High-resolution esophageal manometry study with a 4 cm separation between the LES and crural diaphragm with borderline intact peristaltic contractility. (B) pH impedance on PPI testing with pathologic acid exposure and an elevated number of reflux events. (C) Endoscopic view in forward view (left) and retroflexion (right) of separation between the crural diaphragm and LES.

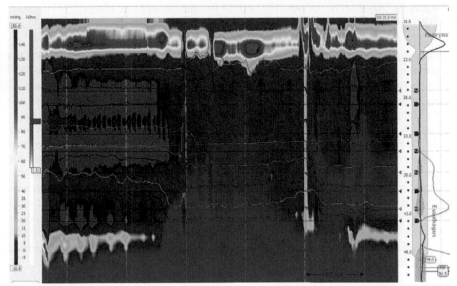

Fig. 4. A TLESR with reflux episode. First, there is inhibition of the crural diaphragm and the LES relaxes for more than 10 seconds; this is accompanied by a gastroesophageal reflux episode.

regarding whether H2RAs help to decrease nocturnal acid breakthrough, studies have shown that in subjects on both double-dose PPI and nightly H2RAs, nighttime reflux symptoms are improved and sleep is less disturbed.[38] Tolerance to H2RAs has been suggested, however, and the benefit of adding H2RAs may wane over time.[39]

Potassium Competitive Acid Blockers

Potassium-competitive acid blockers (P-CABs), such as vonoprazan, competitively inhibit proton pumps and are currently approved in Japan for the treatment of peptic ulcer disease, healing of reflux esophagitis, and eradication of *Helicobacter pylori* infection.[40,41] Compared with PPIs, P-CABs have a higher potency, longer duration of action, and ability to block both inactive and active proton pumps.[32] Multiple retrospective studies have shown a symptomatic improvement in PPI-refractory GERD,[42] and vonoprazan was found to be noninferior to lansoprazole for treatment of erosive esophagitis.[43]

Gamma-Aminobutyric Acid Agonists

Gamma-aminobutyric acid (GABA) agonists, such as Baclofen, have been shown to decrease the number of TLESR events and reduce heartburn and regurgitation symptoms in PPI-refractory GERD when compared with placebo.[44] Potential side effects of GABA agonists, including central nervous system depression, should be considered when selecting patients to start therapy.

Alginate Antacids

Alginate antacids, such as Gaviscon, may be effective in controlling postprandial heartburn and regurgitation.[28,45] When exposed to gastric acid, alginates precipitate and form a floating raft to function as a physical barrier between gastric contents and the LES.[46,47] The low side-effect profile and unique mechanism of action make alginate antacids a helpful adjunct to partial PPI response.[47]

INVASIVE MANAGEMENT OF PROTON PUMP INHIBITOR–REFRACTORY GASTROESOPHAGEAL REFLUX DISEASE

Laparoscopic Fundoplication

Laparoscopic fundoplication involves hernia repair with repositioning of the LES in the intraabdominal cavity and creation of a 1-way flap valve to reduce reflux events.[48–50] Success rates of laparoscopic fundoplication range from 67% to 95% and depend highly on surgical expertise, adequate preoperative evaluation, and appropriate patient selection.[51–53] Nissen fundoplication is a total 360° fundoplication following crural closure. In the setting of impaired esophageal peristaltic reserve at baseline, partial wraps, such as a 270° posterior fundoplication (Toupet) or a 180° anterior fundoplication (Dor), may be preferred to reduce postfundoplication dysphagia.[54] Because the EGJ is a complex anatomic area subject to a multitude of mechanical stresses, the durability of a fundoplication may weaken over time, resulting in hiatal herniation proximal to the wrap and/or slippage of the fundoplication.[55–57] Furthermore, tight fundoplications may result in dysphagia and other obstructive symptoms.[3,24,29] In fact, up to 30% of patients will develop a prolonged structural complication following fundoplication. Additionally, symptoms such as gas-bloat syndrome, chest pain, and diarrhea following fundoplication are common.[58,59]

Magnetic Sphincter Augmentation

Magnetic sphincter augmentation is a new procedure used for treatment of PPI-refractory GERD.[60] This laparoscopic procedure entails placing a magnetic bead device around the LES to augment EGJ pressure through magnetic attraction. In a multicenter trial of 100 subjects, the prevalence of esophagitis after magnetic sphincter augmentation decreased by 28%.[61] In a prospective study of 200 subjects undergoing magnetic sphincter augmentation and repair of large hernias greater than 3 cm, outcomes included postoperative improvement in quality of life.[62] The most common side effect of magnetic sphincter augmentation is dysphagia, and the rate of device migration and esophageal erosion is approximately 0.15%.[63]

Roux-en-Y Gastric Bypass

Obesity is a major risk factor for failure of laparoscopic fundoplication.[64] Procedures such as Roux-en-Y gastric bypass have been studied to treat both GERD and obesity. At 3-year follow-up of 55 subjects with morbid obesity undergoing Roux-en-Y gastric bypass, reflux symptoms improved and incidence of esophagitis decreased.[65] Thus, in the setting of morbid obesity, obesity with related comorbidity, or fundoplication failure, Roux-en-Y gastric bypass should be considered for PPI-refractory GERD.

Transoral Incisionless Fundoplication

Transoral incisionless fundoplication is an endoluminal procedure that aims to reduce hiatal hernia size, restore the physical barrier of the LES, and prevent reflux of gastric contents.[66] In this procedure, a plication device is inserted to first reduce the hiatal hernia and then create a mechanical valve by way of a partial fundoplication.[66,67] In a meta-analysis, transoral incisionless fundoplication did not outperform surgical fundoplication with regard to reduction in esophagitis and increase in LES pressure.[66,68] The rate of serious adverse outcomes, including gastrointestinal perforation and bleeding, was 2.4%.[69]

Radiofrequency Energy Delivery to the Lower Esophageal Sphincter

Another minimally invasive treatment with a low adverse event rate (<1%) improves the barrier function of the EGJ through endoscopic administration of radiofrequency energy to the LES.[70] Studies have shown a significant improvement in symptoms and decreased PPI use with the procedure that applies radiofrequency energy to the LES.[70–76] Nonetheless, concerns of limited postprocedural durability surround both transoral incisionless fundoplication and radiofrequency energy delivery.

SUMMARY

Diagnosis of PPI-refractory GERD requires the presence of troublesome symptoms and objective evidence of ongoing pathologic GERD despite PPI optimization. On PPI therapy, pH-impedance monitoring is the standard method to objectively document PPI-refractory GERD. Alternate causes of PPI nonresponse are common and should be ruled out to avoid misdiagnosis and mismanagement. Mechanisms of PPI-refractory GERD vary and include a dysfunction of protective systems (eg, antireflux barrier, esophageal clearance, epithelial resistance) and enhanced reflux physiology (eg, TLESR episodes, hypotensive LES with free-reflux or strain-induced reflux, re-reflux with hiatal hernia).

As such, management of PPI-refractory GERD should be as tailored to mechanism, patient profile, and patient preference as possible. It is reasonable to switch PPIs from CYP-dependent to less CYP-dependent PPIs (eg, rabeprazole, esomeprazole). H2RAs may be an option for patients reporting nighttime symptoms and/or in the setting of breakthrough nocturnal acid exposure. P-CABs seem to be a promising pharmacologic option for acid-related erosive disease; however, they are not currently available in the United States. GABA agonists, such as Baclofen, may be tried in PPI-refractory GERD, particularly in patients exhibiting TLESRs, an elevated number of reflux events, and regurgitation. GABA agonists may not be as effective in the setting of hiatal hernia. Alginate-antacids carry a favorable safety profile and may be an effective adjunct to PPI.

When noninvasive treatment options fail, invasive antireflux options should be considered. Again, confirmation of objective PPI-refractory GERD is essential because surgical and endoscopic antireflux interventions are associated with risks, and outcomes depend on appropriate patient selection. The gold standard antireflux surgery remains laparoscopic fundoplication in the form of a complete or partial wrap. Other interventions include laparoscopic magnetic sphincter augmentation, endoscopic transoral incisionless fundoplication, or endoscopic radiofrequency energy delivery to the LES. Selection of antireflux intervention requires a discussion of risks and long-term efficacy and durability with the patient.

REFERENCES

1. El-Serag HB, Sweet S, Winchester CC, et al. Update on the epidemiology of gastro-oesophageal reflux disease: a systematic review. Gut 2014;63: 871–80.
2. Peery AF, Crockett SD, Barritt AS, et al. Burden of gastrointestinal, liver, and pancreatic diseases in the United States. Gastroenterology 2015;149:1731–41.e3.
3. Kahrilas PJ, Boeckxstaens G, Smout AJ. Management of the patient with incomplete response to PPI therapy. Best Pract Res Clin Gastroenterol 2013;27:401–14.
4. Yadlapati R, Vaezi MF, Vela MF, et al. Management options for patients with GERD and persistent symptoms on proton pump inhibitors: recommendations from an expert panel. Am J Gastroenterol 2018;113(7):980–6.
5. Kinoshita Y, Hongo M. Efficacy of twice-daily rabeprazole for reflux esophagitis patients refractory to standard once-daily administration of PPI: the Japan-based TWICE study. Am J Gastroenterol 2012;107:522–30.

6. Hsu PI, Lu CL, Wu DC, et al. Eight weeks of esomeprazole therapy reduces symptom relapse, compared with 4 weeks, in patients with Los Angeles grade A or B erosive esophagitis. Clin Gastroenterol Hepatol 2015;13:859–66.e1.
7. Bonavina L, Saino GI, Bona D, et al. Magnetic augmentation of the lower esophageal sphincter: results of a feasibility clinical trial. J Gastrointest Surg 2008;12: 2133–40.
8. Katz PO, Gerson LB, Vela MF. Guidelines for the diagnosis and management of gastroesophageal reflux disease. Am J Gastroenterol 2013;108:308–28 [quiz: 329].
9. Kahrilas PJ, Shaheen NJ, Vaezi MF, et al. American Gastroenterological Association Medical Position Statement on the management of gastroesophageal reflux disease. Gastroenterology 2008;135:1383–91, 1391.e1–5.
10. Vakil N, Niklasson A, Denison H, et al. Symptom profile in partial responders to a proton pump inhibitor compared with treatment-naive patients with gastroesophageal reflux disease: a post hoc analysis of two study populations. BMC Gastroenterol 2014;14:177.
11. Gunaratnam NT, Jessup TP, Inadomi J, et al. Sub-optimal proton pump inhibitor dosing is prevalent in patients with poorly controlled gastro-oesophageal reflux disease. Aliment Pharmacol Ther 2006;23:1473–7.
12. Wolfe MM, Sachs G. Acid suppression: optimizing therapy for gastroduodenal ulcer healing, gastroesophageal reflux disease, and stress-related erosive syndrome. Gastroenterology 2000;118:S9–31.
13. Dean BB, Gano AD Jr, Knight K, et al. Effectiveness of proton pump inhibitors in nonerosive reflux disease. Clin Gastroenterol Hepatol 2004;2:656–64.
14. Roman S, Gyawali CP, Savarino E, et al. Ambulatory reflux monitoring for diagnosis of gastro-esophageal reflux disease: update of the Porto consensus and recommendations from an international consensus group. Neurogastroenterol Motil 2017;29:1–15.
15. Gyawali CP, Roman S, Bredenoord AJ, et al. Classification of esophageal motor findings in gastro-esophageal reflux disease: conclusions from an international consensus group. Neurogastroenterol Motil 2017;29:1–15.
16. Herregods TV, Bredenoord AJ, Smout AJ. Pathophysiology of gastroesophageal reflux disease: new understanding in a new era. Neurogastroenterol Motil 2015; 27:1202–13.
17. Bredenoord AJ, Hemmink GJ, Smout AJ. Relationship between gastro-oesophageal reflux pattern and severity of mucosal damage. Neurogastroenterol Motil 2009;21: 807–12.
18. Anggiansah A, Taylor G, Bright N, et al. Primary peristalsis is the major acid clearance mechanism in reflux patients. Gut 1994;35:1536–42.
19. Kahrilas PJ, Bredenoord AJ, Fox M, et al. The Chicago Classification of esophageal motility disorders, v3.0. Neurogastroenterol Motil 2015;27:160–74.
20. Reddy CA, Patel A, Gyawali CP. Impact of symptom burden and health-related quality of life (HRQOL) on esophageal motor diagnoses. Neurogastroenterol Motil 2017;29:1–8.
21. Tack J, Pandolfino JE. Pathophysiology of gastroesophageal reflux disease. Gastroenterology 2018;154:277–88.
22. Dellon ES, Shaheen NJ. Persistent reflux symptoms in the proton pump inhibitor era: the changing face of gastroesophageal reflux disease. Gastroenterology 2010;139:7–13.e3.
23. Tobey NA, Hosseini SS, Argote CM, et al. Dilated intercellular spaces and shunt permeability in nonerosive acid-damaged esophageal epithelium. Am J Gastroenterol 2004;99:13–22.

24. Kandulski A, Weigt J, Caro C, et al. Esophageal intraluminal baseline impedance differentiates gastroesophageal reflux disease from functional heartburn. Clin Gastroenterol Hepatol 2015;13:1075–81.

25. Ates F, Yuksel ES, Higginbotham T, et al. Mucosal impedance discriminates GERD from non-GERD conditions. Gastroenterology 2015;148:334–43.

26. Emerenziani S, Sifrim D. Gastroesophageal reflux and gastric emptying, revisited. Curr Gastroenterol Rep 2005;7:190–5.

27. Kessing BF, Smout AJ, Bennink RJ, et al. Prucalopride decreases esophageal acid exposure and accelerates gastric emptying in healthy subjects. Neurogastroenterol Motil 2014;26:1079–86.

28. Gyawali CP, Fass R. Management of gastroesophageal reflux disease. Gastroenterology 2018;154:302–18.

29. Ren LH, Chen WX, Qian LJ, et al. Addition of prokinetics to PPI therapy in gastroesophageal reflux disease: a meta-analysis. World J Gastroenterol 2014;20:2412–9.

30. Sifrim D, Castell D, Dent J, et al. Gastro-oesophageal reflux monitoring: review and consensus report on detection and definitions of acid, non-acid, and gas reflux. Gut 2004;53:1024–31.

31. Roman S, Holloway R, Keller J, et al. Validation of criteria for the definition of transient lower esophageal sphincter relaxations using high-resolution manometry. Neurogastroenterol Motil 2017;29:1–9.

32. Hillman L, Yadlapati R, Thuluvath AJ, et al. A review of medical therapy for proton pump inhibitor nonresponsive gastroesophageal reflux disease. Dis Esophagus 2017;30:1–15.

33. Sagar M, Tybring G, Dahl ML, et al. Effects of omeprazole on intragastric pH and plasma gastrin are dependent on the CYP2C19 polymorphism. Gastroenterology 2009;119:670–6.

34. Ishizaki T, Horai Y. Review article: cytochrome P450 and the metabolism of proton pump inhibitors–emphasis on rabeprazole. Aliment Pharmacol Ther 1999;13(Suppl 3):27–36.

35. Furuta T, Ohashi K, Kosuge K, et al. CYP2C19 genotype status and effect of omeprazole on intragastric pH in humans. Clin Pharmacol Ther 1999;65:552–61.

36. Schwab M, Klotz U, Hofmann U, et al. Esomeprazole-induced healing of gastroesophageal reflux disease is unrelated to the genotype of CYP2C19: evidence from clinical and pharmacokinetic data. Clin Pharmacol Ther 2005;78:627–34.

37. Zendehdel N, Biramijamal F, Hossein-Nezhad A, et al. Role of cytochrome P450 2C19 genetic polymorphisms in the therapeutic efficacy of omeprazole in Iranian patients with erosive reflux esophagitis. Arch Iran Med 2010;13:406–12.

38. Rackoff A, Agrawal A, Hila A, et al. Histamine-2 receptor antagonists at night improve gastroesophageal reflux disease symptoms for patients on proton pump inhibitor therapy. Dis Esophagus 2005;18:370–3.

39. Fackler WK, Ours TM, Vaezi MF, et al. Long-term effect of H2RA therapy on nocturnal gastric acid breakthrough. Gastroenterology 2002;122:625–32.

40. Yamashita H, Kanamori A, Kano C, et al. The effects of switching to vonoprazan, a novel potassium-competitive acid blocker, on gastric acidity and reflux patterns in patients with erosive esophagitis refractory to proton pump inhibitors. Digestion 2017;96:52–9.

41. Graham DY, Dore MP. Update on the use of vonoprazan: a competitive acid blocker. Gastroenterology 2018;154:462–6.

42. Shinozaki S, Osawa H, Hayashi Y, et al. Vonoprazan 10 mg daily is effective for the treatment of patients with proton pump inhibitor-resistant gastroesophageal reflux disease. Biomed Rep 2017;7:231–5.

43. Ashida K, Sakurai Y, Hori T, et al. Randomised clinical trial: vonoprazan, a novel potassium-competitive acid blocker, vs. lansoprazole for the healing of erosive oesophagitis. Aliment Pharmacol Ther 2016;43:240–51.

44. Abbasinazari M, Panahi Y, Mortazavi SA, et al. Effect of a combination of omeprazole plus sustained release baclofen versus omeprazole alone on symptoms of patients with gastroesophageal reflux disease (GERD). Iran J Pharm Res 2014; 13:1221–6.

45. Rohof WO, Bennink RJ, Smout AJPM, et al. An alginate-antacid formulation localizes to the acid pocket to reduce acid reflux in patients with gastroesophageal reflux disease. Clin Gastroenterol Hepatol 2013;11:1585–91.

46. Zentilin P, Dulbecco P, Savarino E, et al. An evaluation of the antireflux properties of sodium alginate by means of combined multichannel intraluminal impedance and pH-metry. Aliment Pharmacol Ther 2005;21:29–34.

47. Mandel KG, Daggy BP, Brodie DA, et al. Review article: alginate-raft formulations in the treatment of heartburn and acid reflux. Aliment Pharmacol Ther 2000;14: 669–90.

48. Dallemagne B, Weerts JM, Jehaes C, et al. Laparoscopic Nissen fundoplication: preliminary report. Surg Laparosc Endosc 1991;1:138–43.

49. Geagea T. Laparoscopic Nissen's fundoplication: preliminary report on ten cases. Surg Endosc 1991;5:170–3.

50. Dallemagne B, Weerts J, Markiewicz S, et al. Clinical results of laparoscopic fundoplication at ten years after surgery. Surg Endosc 2006;20:159–65.

51. Jobe BA, Richter JE, Hoppo T, et al. Preoperative diagnostic workup before antireflux surgery: an evidence and experience-based consensus of the Esophageal Diagnostic Advisory Panel. J Am Coll Surg 2013;217:586–97.

52. Fernando HC. Endoscopic fundoplication: patient selection and technique. J Vis Surg 2017;3:121.

53. Moore M, Afaneh C, Benhuri D, et al. Gastroesophageal reflux disease: a review of surgical decision making. World J Gastrointest Surg 2016;8:77–83.

54. Jobe BA, Kahrilas PJ, Vernon AH, et al. Endoscopic appraisal of the gastroesophageal valve after antireflux surgery. Am J Gastroenterol 2004;99:233–43.

55. Richter JE. Let the patient beware: the evolving truth about laparoscopic antireflux surgery. Am J Med 2003;114:71–3.

56. Hinder RA, Libbey JS, Gorecki P, et al. Antireflux surgery. Indications, preoperative evaluation, and outcome. Gastroenterol Clin North Am 1999;28:987–1005, viii.

57. Horgan S, Pohl D, Bogetti D, et al. Failed antireflux surgery: what have we learned from reoperations? Arch Surg 1999;134:809–15 [discussion: 815–7].

58. Swanstrom L, Wayne R. Spectrum of gastrointestinal symptoms after laparoscopic fundoplication. Am J Surg 1994;167:538–41.

59. Lundell L. Complications after anti-reflux surgery. Best Pract Res Clin Gastroenterol 2004;18:935–45.

60. Buckley FP 3rd, Bell RCW, Freeman K, et al. Favorable results from a prospective evaluation of 200 patients with large hiatal hernias undergoing LINX magnetic sphincter augmentation. Surg Endosc 2018;32(4):1762–8.

61. Azagury D, Morton J. Surgical anti-reflux options beyond fundoplication. Curr Gastroenterol Rep 2017;19:35.

62. Buckley FP 3rd, Bell RCW, Freeman K, et al. Favorable results from a prospective evaluation of 200 patients with large hiatal hernias undergoing LINX magnetic sphincter augmentation. Surg Endosc 2018;32:1762–8.
63. Smith CD, Ganz RA, Lipham JC, et al. Lower esophageal sphincter augmentation for gastroesophageal reflux disease: the safety of a modern implant. J Laparoendosc Adv Surg Tech A 2017;27:586–91.
64. Perez AR, Moncure AC, Rattner DW. Obesity adversely affects the outcome of antireflux operations. Surg Endosc 2001;15:986–9.
65. Madalosso CA, Gurski RR, Callegari-Jacques SM, et al. The impact of gastric bypass on gastroesophageal reflux disease in morbidly obese patients. Ann Surg 2016;263:110–6.
66. Richter JE, Kumar A, Lipka S, et al. Efficacy of laparoscopic Nissen fundoplication vs transoral incisionless fundoplication or proton pump inhibitors in patients with gastroesophageal reflux disease: a systematic review and network meta-analysis. Gastroenterology 2018;154(5):1298–308.e7.
67. Hakansson B, Montgomery M, Cadiere GB, et al. Randomised clinical trial: transoral incisionless fundoplication vs. sham intervention to control chronic GERD. Aliment Pharmacol Ther 2015;42:1261–70.
68. Trad KS, Barnes WE, Prevou ER, et al. The TEMPO trial at 5 years: transoral fundoplication (TIF 2.0) is safe, durable, and cost-effective. Surg Innov 2018;25(2):149–57.
69. Huang X, Chen S, Zhao H, et al. Efficacy of transoral incisionless fundoplication (TIF) for the treatment of GERD: a systematic review with meta-analysis. Surg Endosc 2017;31:1032–44.
70. Franciosa M, Mashimo H. Stretta radiofrequency treatment for GERD: a safe and effective modality. Am J Gastroenterol 2013;108:1654–5.
71. Kim MS, Dent J, Holloway RH, et al. Radiofrequency energy delivery to the gastric cardia inhibits triggering of transient lower esophageal sphincter relaxation in a canine model. Gastroenterology;118:A860.
72. Arts J, Bisschops R, Blondeau K, et al. A double-blind sham-controlled study of the effect of radiofrequency energy on symptoms and distensibility of the gastroesophageal junction in GERD. Am J Gastroenterol 2012;107:222–30.
73. Arts J, Sifrim D, Rutgeerts P, et al. Influence of radiofrequency energy delivery at the gastroesophageal junction (the Stretta procedure) on symptoms, acid exposure, and esophageal sensitivity to acid perfusion in gastroesophagal reflux disease. Dig Dis Sci 2007;52:2170–7.
74. Triadafilopoulos G, DiBaise JK, Nostrant TT, et al. The Stretta procedure for the treatment of GERD: 6 and 12 month follow-up of the U.S. open label trial. Gastrointest Endosc 2002;55:149–56.
75. Sifrim D, Zerbib F. Diagnosis and management of patients with reflux symptoms refractory to proton pump inhibitors. Gut 2012;61:1340–54.
76. Fass R, Cahn F, Scotti DJ, et al. Systematic review and meta-analysis of controlled and prospective cohort efficacy studies of endoscopic radiofrequency for treatment of gastroesophageal reflux disease. Surg Endosc 2017;31:4865–82.

Eosinophilic Esophagitis

Craig C. Reed, MD, MSCR[a], Evan S. Dellon, MD, MPH[b],*

KEYWORDS

- Eosinophilic esophagitis • Dysphagia • Food bolus impaction • Heartburn

KEY POINTS

- Eosinophilic esophagitis has emerged as an important contributor to upper gastrointestinal morbidity.
- Primary care providers are indispensable for the timely and accurate diagnosis of eosinophilic esophagitis.
- A delay in diagnosis of eosinophilic esophagitis contributes to the risk of long-term complications.

INTRODUCTION

Eosinophilic esophagitis (EoE) is a chronic disorder characterized clinically by symptoms of esophageal dysfunction and histologically by eosinophilic infiltration of the esophageal epithelium.[1–3] The disease belongs to the spectrum of eosinophilic gastrointestinal disorders whereby eosinophilic inflammation of the gastrointestinal tract occurs in the absence of secondary causes. Before the 1990s when esophageal eosinophilia was thought to be solely due to reflux esophagitis,[4] EoE was rarely recognized. However, by the mid-1990s, seminal papers described the condition,[5] and the number of publications on EoE increased dramatically.[6] EoE represents an important contributor to upper gastrointestinal morbidity throughout the world, a growing health problem, and a significant burden for health care systems.[7,8]

Financial Support: This research was funded by NIH Awards T32 DK007634 (C.C. Reed) and R01 DK101856 (E.S. Dellon).
Potential Competing Interests: Neither of the authors reports any potential conflicts of interest with this article. Dr E.S. Dellon is a consultant for Adare, Alivio, Banner, Enumeral, GSK, Receptos/Celegene, Regeneron, and Shire; receives research funding from Adare, Meritage, Miraca, Nutricia, Receptos/Celgene, Regeneron, and Shire; and has received educational grants from Banner and Holoclara.

a Division of Gastroenterology and Hepatology, Department of Medicine, Center for Esophageal Diseases and Swallowing, Center for Gastrointestinal Biology and Disease, University of North Carolina School of Medicine, 130 Mason Farm Road, Chapel Hill, NC 27599-7080, USA;
b Division of Gastroenterology and Hepatology, Department of Medicine, Center for Esophageal Diseases and Swallowing, Center for Gastrointestinal Biology and Disease, University of North Carolina School of Medicine, CB #7080, Room 4140, Bioinformatics Building, 130 Mason Farm Road, Chapel Hill, NC 27599-7080, USA
* Corresponding author.
E-mail address: edellon@med.unc.edu

Med Clin N Am 103 (2019) 29–42
https://doi.org/10.1016/j.mcna.2018.08.009
0025-7125/19/© 2018 Elsevier Inc. All rights reserved.

Important roles exist across medical specialties for the comanagement of EoE. This includes primary care providers, allergists, gastroenterologists, pathologists, and nutritionists treating both adult and pediatric patients. For the primary care provider, the identification and referral of patients with suspected EoE is indispensable. Despite the increase in EoE-pertinent literature, patients endorse a protracted diagnostic delay following symptom initiation. Furthermore, this delay has yet to decrease and correlates with prognosis.[1,9] Primary care providers are thus pivotal not only for timely and accurate diagnosis, but also to recognize the existence of comorbid conditions and to initiate specialist referrals.[2]

This article aims to provide the critical information necessary to facilitate the incorporation of primary care providers into the comanagement of EoE. To achieve this, we provide an overview of EoE clinical, endoscopic, and histologic features as well as treatment options and future directions in management.

CLINICAL PRESENTATION
Symptoms Reported by Patients with Eosinophilic Esophagitis

The diagnosis of EoE starts with a thorough investigation of presenting symptoms. These vary by patient age (**Table 1**).

Practitioners should consider EoE in adolescents and adults when the predominant complaint is esophageal dysphagia,[10] which is reported by 60% to 100% of patients,[6,11,12] and food impaction can be seen in more than 25%.[13,14] Heartburn (30%–60%) and noncardiac chest pain (8%–44%) are commonly reported,[11,15] and EoE may be present in 1% to 8% of patients with proton pump inhibitor (PPI) refractory reflux symptoms.[16,17] Abdominal pain, nausea, vomiting, diarrhea, gastrointestinal bleeding, and weight loss are uncharacteristic in adults with EoE, and a different process or more diffuse eosinophilic gastrointestinal disorder (eg, eosinophilic gastroenteritis, eosinophilic colitis) should be considered when these features predominate.

Children with EoE report nonspecific complaints (see **Table 1**).[18] Difficulty feeding, choking, refusal of food, and vomiting are also found in infants and toddlers.[19,20] When constitutional symptoms, such as fever and weight loss predominate, an alternative disease should be sought.

Elucidating symptoms of dysphagia can be a subtle task, as many patients have subconsciously developed compensatory eating behaviors over years to minimize symptoms. Specific behaviors to assess include the following:

- Eating slowly
- Excessive food chewing
- Lubrication of food boluses or drinking a copious amount of liquid after each bite
- Repeated swallows to facilitate food bolus passage
- Avoidance of troublesome foods
- Crushing or avoiding pills

Table 1 Common symptoms associated with eosinophilic esophagitis	
Adolescents and Adults	**Children**
Solid food dysphagia	Nausea and vomiting
Food bolus impaction	Regurgitation
Heartburn	Heartburn
Chest pain	Abdominal pain
	Chest pain
	Anorexia/feeding refusal/failure to thrive

Comorbid Conditions Associated with Eosinophilic Esophagitis

Atopy is commonly encountered in EoE cohorts, and for adult EoE patients, the prevalence of any atopic condition is 20% to 80%.[12] Children with EoE have a prevalence of 30% to 50% and 50% to 75% for asthma and allergic rhinitis, which compares with 10% to 30% for either condition in the general pediatric population. Furthermore, children with EoE are more likely to develop environmental allergies and immunoglobulin (Ig)E-mediated food allergy (eg, urticaria, anaphylaxis).[21,22] Moreover, a family history of an atopic disorder is found in more than 50% of patients with EoE.[23]

EoE also develops in association with some genetic syndromes, including inherited connective tissue disorders that exhibit hypermobility.[24,25] However, this is rare and only 1% of patients with EoE present with this phenotype.

Familial Susceptibility to Eosinophilic Esophagitis

Although EoE does not demonstrate classic Mendelian inheritance, there is a genetic component,[26] and a familial history of EoE increases individual risk for the condition above the approximately 1 of 2000 seen in the general population (see the epidemiology section, later in this article). The risk varies by the particular relationship[19]:

- Any first-degree relative: 1.8% individual risk (recurrence risk ratio: 33)
- Father: 2.4% individual risk (recurrence risk ratio: 43)
- Mother: 0.6% individual risk (recurrence risk ratio: 10)
- Brother: 3.5% individual risk (recurrence risk ratio: 64)
- Sister: 1.3% individual risk (recurrence risk ratio: 24)[27]

There is also significant concordance for EoE in both monozygotic (40%) and dizygotic twins (30%). The latter findings implicate the role of early-life exposures in EoE susceptibility.[27]

Endoscopic Findings Common to Eosinophilic Esophagitis

Multiple, though nonspecific,[28] structural changes of the esophagus are seen with EoE,[2] and these can vary by patient age.[11] Fibrostenotic findings, such as esophageal rings, strictures, or narrowing are more common in adults, whereas inflammatory findings, such as white plaques/exudates, linear furrows, and edema/decreased vascularity are more common in children (**Fig. 1**). Although all findings can be seen across the age spectrum, the difference in findings by age is thought to reflect a fibrotic esophageal response to chronic eosinophilic inflammation.[29–31] Other findings include a diffusely narrowed or small-caliber esophagus,[32,33] and crepe-paper mucosa (eg, tearing of the esophageal mucosa from passage of an endoscope). Endoscopic findings of EoE are frequently described using the EoE endoscopic reference score (EREFS), which stands for the 5 key findings of Edema, Rings, Exudates, Furrows, and Strictures.[34] This system provides greater uniformity in the description of findings, identifies and discriminates between patients with and without EoE, and correlates with treatment.[35,36]

Histologic Features of Eosinophilic Esophagitis

All patients exhibit increased intraepithelial eosinophils that may be found in all regions of the esophagus (**Fig. 2**). Eosinophil surface layering and eosinophilic microabscesses, dilated intercellular spaces, a thickened mucosa with basal layer hyperplasia and papillary elongation, and extracellular deposition of eosinophil granule proteins, such as eosinophil peroxidase are also found.[37,38] Patients with fibrostenotic complications of EoE (eg, rings, strictures) exhibit increased collagen deposition within the lamina propria.[39]

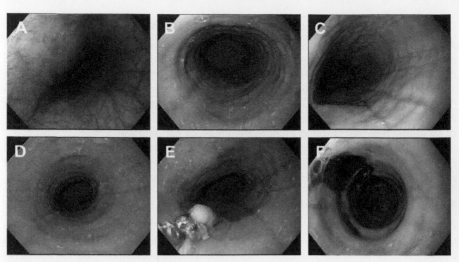

Fig. 1. Endoscopic images of EoE. (*A*) The endoscopic appearance of the normal esophagus. Note the uniform and smooth appearance of the esophageal mucosa, with the fine vascular pattern clearly visible. (*B*) A patient with EoE with evidence of esophageal rings, furrows, edema, and exudates. (*C*) A patient with EoE with esophageal edema, deep furrows, and mild exudates. (*D*) A patient with EoE with a focal stricture, in addition to mild rings, furrows, edema, and exudates. (*E*) Esophageal biopsy under way. (*F*) A patient with EoE with a very narrow caliber esophagus and tight rings, as well as edema, after esophageal dilation. Good dilation effect (mucosal rent) is seen in the 11 o'clock position (H&E stain).

DIAGNOSTIC CRITERIA
Diagnostic Criteria and Consensus Guidelines Definition

EoE is a chronic immune and antigen-mediated *clinicopathologic* disease,[1–3] and diagnostic criteria require both the appropriate clinical and histologic features:

- Symptoms of esophageal dysfunction (see **Table 1**)
- Presence of esophageal eosinophilia with a peak of at least 15 eosinophils in a high-power microscopy field (eos/hpf)
- Exclusion of alternative etiologies of esophageal eosinophilia[1]

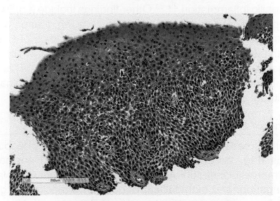

Fig. 2. Histologic image of an esophageal biopsy in EoE. In addition to the prominent eosinophilic infiltration (>15 eos/hpf), there is eosinophil degranulation, basal zone hyperplasia, and spongiosis.

Although initially selected by expert opinion, the threshold of 15 eos/hpf achieves a sensitivity of 100% and a specificity of 96% for establishing the diagnosis.[40] It is worth noting that patients with lower levels of eosinophilia and phenotypic features have been reported, and they may have EoE in appropriate settings.[41]

With regard to the third criterion stipulated previously, previous guidelines[1] required nonresponse to a PPI trial to establish the diagnosis. Patients responding to PPI were labeled with PPI-responsive esophageal eosinophilia (PPI-REE), which became an area of substantial controversy.[42] However, this distinction is no longer required, and PPIs have evolved from a diagnostic tool to a treatment option.[3]

Alternative Etiologies of Esophageal Eosinophilia

Esophageal eosinophilia is not pathognomonic for EoE. Alternative etiologies should be sought and ruled out following a thorough history, physical examination, and select laboratory tests. The most prevalent competing or overlapping diagnosis is gastroesophageal reflux disease (GERD). Less common competing diagnoses include the following[1-3]:

- Achalasia
- Infection
- Connective tissue diseases
- Crohn disease
- Pill esophagitis
- Hypereosinophilic syndrome
- Drug hypersensitivity[1-3]

When more generalized eosinophilic infiltration of the gastrointestinal tract is noted, the findings may be consistent with eosinophilic gastroenteritis and/or colitis with esophageal involvement.

Because GERD can induce EoE and produces similar symptoms to EoE, the differentiation of the 2 conditions proves challenging.[43] Complicating this matter, the relationship between GERD and EoE remains controversial. For instance, GERD and EoE may simply overlap, EoE may induce GERD through impaired esophageal clearance of refluxate, or GERD may conceivably cause EoE by damaging the epithelial border and thus allow for the presentation of antigens and a subsequent allergic response.[44] Altogether, symptoms of reflux should be sought and treated, and pH monitoring has not successfully discriminated GERD from EoE.[45]

EPIDEMIOLOGY

EoE is found globally. Many cases have been reported in North America, South America, Europe, and Australia. Cases also exist from Asia and the Middle East. India and Sub-Saharan Africa are exceptional, with no cases documented from these areas.[46] EoE is more common in cold and arid climates, and in rural areas,[47] and most frequently affects those younger than 50,[48] men, and Caucasians.[7]

According to data derived largely from North American and European cohorts, the pooled incidence rate of EoE is 3.7 per 100,000 patient years (95% confidence interval 1.7–6.5).[49] Additionally, all studies examining EoE incidence have found an increasing incidence over time[50] not explained by disease awareness or utilization of endoscopy.[11] Similarly, prevalence data estimated an overall pooled prevalence of 22.7 per 100,000 (95% confidence interval 12.4–36.0),[49] and this value has also increased over time.[7]

The aforementioned changes in EoE incidence and prevalence suggest that environmental factors, as opposed to genetic factors, drive the changing epidemiology,[46] but the exact etiology is not known. Early-life exposures, including antibiotic use in infancy, cesarean delivery, preterm birth, and lack of breastfeeding, have been implicated as disease risk factors.[27,51] It has been hypothesized that these factors may affect the microbiome and the developing immune system. In addition, decreased *Helicobacter pylori* prevalence, increased PPI use, changes in food sources, and food packaging have also been implicated in the changing epidemiology of EoE.[7]

PATHOGENESIS

Animal models, genetic studies, comorbid allergic disorders, and the efficacy of elimination diets suggest that EoE is an atopic condition.[26] Most patients are sensitive to 1 or more foods[52] and have aeroallergen hypersensitivity[2] or respiratory allergy.[53] Similarly, the role of antigen sensitization is supported by clinical and histologic improvements with elimination diets devoid of precipitating allergens.[54] Mounting data show that EoE is not IgE-mediated[55] and IgG4 may have a role in disease pathogenesis.[55]

EoE is also Th2-mediated. Th2 cells produce inflammatory cytokines, including interleukin (IL)-4, IL-5, and IL-13 that in turn increase eotaxin-3. The latter molecule is a potent chemokine inducing eosinophilic infiltration into and activation within the esophagus.[56] Once activated, eosinophils produce additional factors, such as transforming growth factor (TGF)-beta. TGF-beta promotes tissue remodeling of the esophagus that contributes to the fibrostenotic complications of EoE.[57,58]

TREATMENTS

Drugs, *diet*, and *dilation* encapsulate the treatment paradigms for EoE.[59] Drugs and diet reduce EoE-associated inflammation and dilation targets esophageal strictures and narrowing. Treatment choice is predicated on patient preference, clinical features, and cost. Goals of therapy include clinical and histologic improvement and reduction in long-term complications. No Food and Drug Administration–approved medication exists for EoE, and as such, all medications are used off label in the United States. Many patients with EoE will continue to be followed by their primary care provider, so it is important to be familiar with EoE treatment options, even if these are initially directed by specialists.

PPIs are an initial pharmacologic choice for EoE. If PPI nonresponse occurs (**Fig. 3**), corticosteroids or elimination diet are used. Treatment should be optimized and factors associated with response (eg, adherence, drug dose, inadvertent antigen exposure, esophageal infection, stricture) assessed at each follow-up visit.[60]

Corticosteroids, whether delivered topically or systemically, improve the clinical symptoms and histologic features of EoE. Systemic corticosteroids are now reserved for patients requiring a prompt therapeutic response, such as severe symptoms or growth failure, owing to their long-term adverse effects as well as the results of a randomized controlled trial (RCT) illustrating similar efficacy of topical and systemic corticosteroids.[61] Methods for delivering topical corticosteroids include swallowing fluticasone (puffed into the mouth from an asthma multidose inhaler [MDI] and then swallowed) or budesonide (mixed in a viscous slurry from the aqueous asthma nebulizer formulation).

The decision to use an elimination diet depends on multiple factors:

- Acceptability of the diet by patient and family
- Provider expertise
- Availability of dieticians

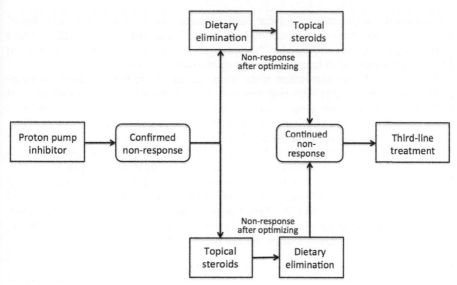

Fig. 3. Treatment algorithm for the primary and secondary treatment of eosinophilic esophagitis.

Types of elimination diets include elemental liquid amino acid–based formulations,[62] empiric elimination diets,[54,63] and allergy test–directed diets.[64–66]

Efficacy of Pharmacologic and Dietary Treatment Strategies

Studies analyzing adults and children illustrated that between 33% and 74% of patients with EoE respond to PPIs.[45,67] Moreover, a meta-analysis documented a pooled PPI response rate of approximately 50%.[68] The long-term efficacy of PPIs is less clear. A recent prospective study documented that most pediatric patients (78%) remain in clinical and histologic remission following 1 year of maintenance therapy,[69] and similar data are available for adults.[70] In addition, temporary discontinuation of PPI therapy results in recurrence of symptoms and/or histologic relapse. However, PPI reintroduction recaptures response in most patients.

Topical corticosteroid efficacy has been well studied in multiple RCTs, and several meta-analyses summarize their data.[71,72] They have consistently produced reductions in esophageal eosinophil counts versus comparator and are capable of maintaining remission in a proportion of patients. The typical doses used for oral viscous budesonide as well as fluticasone in clinical trials are summarized in **Table 2**.

Correct techniques must be stressed to optimize esophageal deposition of topical corticosteroids. Topical corticosteroids should be taken following meals and patients should avoid eating or drinking for 30 to 60 minutes after swallowing the medication. Additionally, MDIs are ideally administered at end expiration following a breath hold.

Table 2		
Typical doses of topical corticosteroids for eosinophilic esophagitis		
Topical Corticosteroid	**Age**	**Dose**
Fluticasone via multidose inhaler	Children	440–880 µg/d
	Adults and adolescents	880–1760 µg/d
Oral viscous budesonide	Children	1 mg/d
	Adults and adolescents	2–4 mg/d

A common complication of topical corticosteroid use is esophageal candidiasis, which is seen on follow-up endoscopy in 10% to 20% of patients with EoE.[73] A rare complication is herpes esophagitis.[74] Additionally, a recent systematic review noted that adrenal suppression following topical corticosteroids is uncommon.[75]

The efficacy of food elimination diets varies according to the diet used. A meta-analysis of adult patients with EoE reported that elemental diets were effective in 91%, empiric elimination diets in 72%, and allergy test–directed diets in 46%.[64] Elemental diets produce histologic remission in most patients. However, practical limitations limit their use (eg, cost, palatability, gastrostomy tube placement, quality of life).[1] Conversely, allergy test–directed diets produce lower rates of remission as a consequence of their low predictive value for the identification of culprit foods.[54,76] Empiric diets have thus become the elimination strategy of choice. The most common and best described is the "6-food elimination diet" that removes dairy, wheat, egg, soy, peanut/tree nut, and fish/shellfish. For patients undergoing dietary elimination, working with a nutritionist or dietician is recommended to help increase compliance, decrease inadvertent contamination, and prevent nutritional deficiencies.[77]

The Role of Esophageal Dilation in Eosinophilic Esophagitis

Esophageal stricture or narrowing is treated best by dilation, which is safe and effective when done cautiously. This is an important treatment to improve symptoms of dysphagia, but it does not impact the underlying eosinophilic inflammation.[78] A meta-analysis determined a 0.3% risk for perforation, although at expert centers, and this value is comparable to the risk of perforation following dilation of patients without EoE.[79]

FUTURE DIRECTIONS

Future directions in the management of EoE pertain to diagnosis and follow-up, topical corticosteroid formulations, and novel treatments. Researchers are actively seeking less invasive and more efficient diagnostic tools (eg, tethered capsule endoscopy, unsedated transnasal endoscopy, cytosponge-obtained esophageal tissue collection, or string-based analysis of esophageal inflammatory factors).[80–83] Genetic features may also assist in the diagnosis of EoE: the EoE transcriptome may accurately identify the disease[84] and assist in predicting clinical outcomes.[85] Serum biomarkers are of intense interest, but to date none have been found to be ready for clinical use.[86,87]

New formulations for topical corticosteroid delivery are under study. An effervescent budesonide tablet was highly effective as a means of delivery in an RCT,[88] and has been recommended for approval for EoE in Europe. Another RCT found pre-prepared viscous budesonide to be both safe and effective and capable of inducing clinical, endoscopic, and histologic remission.[89]

Small molecules including angiotensin receptor blockers (eg, losartan) (NCT01808196), Janus kinase inhibitors,[90] and OCT000459,[91] an oral drug that blocks the effects of prostaglandin D2, are emerging as potential treatment options and have been studied to varying degrees. Biologic agents, including anti–IL-5 monoclonal antibodies (which are approved for eosinophilic asthma),[92–94] anti–IL-13 antibodies,[95,96] and the anti–IL-4r blocker dupilumab (which has recently been approved for eczema),[97] are also under study. The place of these biologics in the treatment algorithm for EoE has yet to be determined.

In addition to the aforementioned future directions, health care transition from pediatric-focused to adult-focused systems represents an important and under-studied topic.[98] In one study, most patients and parents of children with EoE were found to be unfamiliar with health care transition. Readiness for transition was also low compared with other chronic diseases.[99] As such, exploration of barriers limiting transition readiness should be a priority, especially in light of the large cohort of patients with EoE transitioning to adult care, and coordination of this care transition is another role for primary care providers.

SUMMARY

EoE is a chronic disorder characterized by symptoms of esophageal dysfunction and esophageal inflammation with intraepithelial eosinophils. EoE represents an important global contributor to gastrointestinal morbidity. Primary care providers are pivotal for timely and accurate detection of symptoms potentially related to EoE, referral to proper specialists for diagnosis, coordination of care between multiple providers, as well as transition of care from pediatric to adult providers, all with the goal of improving patient quality of life and reducing long-term EoE complications.

REFERENCES

1. Dellon ES, Gonsalves N, Hirano I, et al. ACG clinical guideline: evidenced based approach to the diagnosis and management of esophageal eosinophilia and eosinophilic esophagitis (EoE). Am J Gastroenterol 2013;108(5):679–92.
2. Liacouras CA, Furuta GT, Hirano I, et al. Eosinophilic esophagitis: updated consensus recommendations for children and adults. J Allergy Clin Immunol 2011;128(1):3–20.
3. Lucendo AJ, Molina-Infante J, Arias Á, et al. Guidelines on eosinophilic esophagitis: evidence-based statements and recommendations for diagnosis and management in children and adults. United European Gastroenterol J 2017;5(3): 335–58.
4. Winter HS, Madara JL, Stafford RJ, et al. Intraepithelial eosinophils: a new diagnostic criterion for reflux esophagitis. Gastroenterology 1982;83(4):818–23.
5. Attwood SEA, Smyrk TC, Demeester TR, et al. Esophageal eosinophilia with dysphagia—a distinct clinicopathologic syndrome. Dig Dis Sci 1993;38(1): 109–16.
6. Dellon ES, Aderoju A, Woosley JT, et al. Variability in diagnostic criteria for eosinophilic esophagitis: a systematic review. Am J Gastroenterol 2007;102(10): 2300–13.
7. Dellon ES, Hirano I. Epidemiology and natural history of eosinophilic esophagitis. Gastroenterology 2017;154(2):319–32.
8. Jensen ET, Kappelman MD, Martin CF, et al. Health-care utilization, costs, and the burden of disease related to eosinophilic esophagitis in the United States. Am J Gastroenterol 2015;110(5):626–32.
9. Reed CC, Koutlas NT, Robey BS, et al. Prolonged time to diagnosis of eosinophilic esophagitis despite increasing knowledge of the disease. Clin Gastroenterol Hepatol 2018. https://doi.org/10.1016/j.cgh.2018.01.028.
10. Dellon ES, Kim HP, Sperry SLW, et al. A phenotypic analysis shows that eosinophilic esophagitis is a progressive fibrostenotic disease. Gastrointest Endosc 2014;79(4):577–85.
11. Dellon ES, Gibbs WB, Fritchie KJ, et al. Clinical, endoscopic, and histologic findings distinguish eosinophilic esophagitis from gastroesophageal reflux disease. Clin Gastroenterol Hepatol 2009;7(12):1305–13.
12. Dellon ES, Liacouras CA. Advances in clinical management of eosinophilic esophagitis. Gastroenterology 2014;147(6):1238–54.

13. Sperry SLW, Crockett SD, Miller CB, et al. Esophageal foreign-body impactions: epidemiology, time trends, and the impact of the increasing prevalence of eosinophilic esophagitis. Gastrointest Endosc 2011;74(5):985–91.
14. Hiremath GS, Hameed F, Pacheco A, et al. Esophageal food impaction and eosinophilic esophagitis: a retrospective study, systematic review, and meta-analysis. Dig Dis Sci 2015;60(11):3181–93.
15. Gonsalves N, Policarpio-Nicolas M, Zhang Q, et al. Histopathologic variability and endoscopic correlates in adults with eosinophilic esophagitis. Gastrointest Endosc 2006;64(3):313–9.
16. Veerappan GR, Perry JL, Duncan TJ, et al. Prevalence of eosinophilic esophagitis in an adult population undergoing upper endoscopy: a prospective study. Clin Gastroenterol Hepatol 2009;7(4):420–6.
17. Dellon ES, Speck O, Woodward K, et al. Clinical and endoscopic characteristics do not reliably differentiate PPI-responsive esophageal eosinophilia and eosinophilic esophagitis in patients undergoing upper endoscopy: a prospective cohort study. Am J Gastroenterol 2013;108(12):1854–60.
18. Liacouras CA, Spergel JM, Ruchelli E, et al. Eosinophilic esophagitis: a 10-year experience in 381 children. Clin Gastroenterol Hepatol 2005;3(12):1198–206.
19. Noel RJ, Putnam PE, Rothenberg ME. Eosinophilic esophagitis. N Engl J Med 2004;351(9):940–1.
20. Liacouras CA, Markowitz JE. Eosinophilic esophagitis: a subset of eosinophilic gastroenteritis. Curr Gastroenterol Rep 1999;1:253–8.
21. Simon D, Marti H, Heer P, et al. Eosinophilic esophagitis is frequently associated with IgE-mediated allergic airway diseases. J Allergy Clin Immunol 2005;115(5): 1090–2.
22. Assa'ad AH, Putnam PE, Collins MH, et al. Pediatric patients with eosinophilic esophagitis: an 8-year follow-up. J Allergy Clin Immunol 2007;119(3):731–8.
23. Assa'ad A. Eosinophilic esophagitis: association with allergic disorders. Gastrointest Endosc Clin N Am 2008;18(1):119–32.
24. Frischmeyer-Guerrerio PA, Guerrerio AL, Oswald G, et al. Allergy: TGFβ receptor mutations impose a strong predisposition for human allergic disease. Sci Transl Med 2013;5(195):195ra94.
25. Abonia JP, Wen T, Stucke EM, et al. High prevalence of eosinophilic esophagitis in patients with inherited connective tissue disorders. J Allergy Clin Immunol 2013;132(2):378–86.
26. O'Shea K, Aceves S, Dellon E, et al. Pathophysiology of eosinophilic esophagitis. Gastroenterology 2018;154(2):333–45.
27. Alexander ES, Martin LJ, Collins MH, et al. Twin and family studies reveal strong environmental and weaker genetic cues explaining heritability of eosinophilic esophagitis. J Allergy Clin Immunol 2014;134(5):1084–92.
28. Kim HP, Vance RB, Shaheen NJ, et al. The prevalence and diagnostic utility of endoscopic features of eosinophilic esophagitis: a meta-analysis. Clin Gastroenterol Hepatol 2012;10(9):988–96.
29. Aceves SS, Newbury RO, Chen D, et al. Resolution of remodeling in eosinophilic esophagitis correlates with epithelial response to topical corticosteroids. Allergy 2010;65(1):109–16.
30. Schoepfer AM, Safroneeva E, Bussmann C, et al. Delay in diagnosis of eosinophilic esophagitis increases risk for stricture formation in a time-dependent manner. Gastroenterology 2013;145(6):1230–6.
31. Koutlas NT, Dellon ES. Progression from an inflammatory to a fibrostenotic phenotype in eosinophilic esophagitis. Case Rep Gastroenterol 2017;11(2):382–8.

32. Lee J, Huprich J, Kujath C, et al. Esophageal diameter is decreased in some patients with eosinophilic esophagitis and might increase with topical corticosteroid therapy. Clin Gastroenterol Hepatol 2012;10(5):481–6.

33. Eluri S, Runge TM, Cotton CC, et al. The extremely narrow-caliber esophagus is a treatment-resistant subphenotype of eosinophilic esophagitis. Gastrointest Endosc 2016;83(6):1142–8.

34. Hirano I, Moy N, Heckman MG, et al. Endoscopic assessment of the oesophageal features of eosinophilic oesophagitis: validation of a novel classification and grading system. Gut 2013;62(4):489–95.

35. Dellon ES, Cotton CC, Gebhart JH, et al. Accuracy of the eosinophilic esophagitis endoscopic reference score in diagnosis and determining response to treatment. Clin Gastroenterol Hepatol 2016;14(1):31–9.

36. Wechsler J, Bolton S, Amsden K, et al. Eosinophilic esophagitis reference score accurately identifies disease activity and treatment effects in children. Clin Gastroenterol Hepatol 2018;16(7):1056–63.

37. Protheroe C, Woodruff SA, de Petris G, et al. A novel histologic scoring system to evaluate mucosal biopsies from patients with eosinophilic esophagitis. Clin Gastroenterol Hepatol 2009;7(7):749–55.

38. Collins MH. Histopathologic features of eosinophilic esophagitis and eosinophilic gastrointestinal diseases. Gastroenterol Clin North Am 2014;43(2):257–68.

39. Aceves SS. Tissue remodeling in patients with eosinophilic esophagitis: what lies beneath the surface? J Allergy Clin Immunol 2011;128(5):1047–9.

40. Dellon S, Speck O, Woodward K, et al. Distribution and variability of esophageal eosinophilia in patients undergoing upper endoscopy. Mod Pathol 2015;28(3):383–90.

41. Ravi K, Talley NJ, Smyrk TC, et al. Low grade esophageal eosinophilia in adults: an unrecognized part of the spectrum of eosinophilic esophagitis? Dig Dis Sci 2011;56(7):1981–6.

42. Molina-Infante J, Bredenoord AJ, Cheng E, et al. Proton pump inhibitor-responsive oesophageal eosinophilia: an entity challenging current diagnostic criteria for eosinophilic oesophagitis. Gut 2016;65(3):521–31.

43. Rodrigo S, Abboud G, Oh D, et al. High intraepithelial eosinophil counts in esophageal squamous epithelium are not specific for eosinophilic esophagitis in adults. Am J Gastroenterol 2008;103(2):435–42.

44. Spechler SJ, Genta RM, Souza RF. Thoughts on the complex relationship between gastroesophageal reflux disease and eosinophilic esophagitis. Am J Gastroenterol 2007;102(6):1301–6.

45. Francis DL, Foxx-Orenstein A, Arora AS, et al. Results of ambulatory pH monitoring do not reliably predict response to therapy in patients with eosinophilic oesophagitis. Aliment Pharmacol Ther 2012;35(2):300–7.

46. Dellon ES. Epidemiology of eosinophilic esophagitis. Gastroenterol Clin North Am 2014;43(2):201–18.

47. Jensen ET, Hoffman K, Shaheen NJ, et al. Esophageal eosinophilia is increased in rural areas with low population density: results from a national pathology database. Am J Gastroenterol 2014;109(5):668–75.

48. Dellon ES, Jensen ET, Martin CF, et al. Prevalence of eosinophilic esophagitis in the United States. Clin Gastroenterol Hepatol 2014;12(4):589–96.

49. Arias Á, Pérez-Martínez I, Tenías JM, et al. Systematic review with meta-analysis: the incidence and prevalence of eosinophilic oesophagitis in children and adults in population-based studies. Aliment Pharmacol Ther 2016;43(1):3–15.

50. Prasad GA, Alexander JA, Schleck CD, et al. Epidemiology of eosinophilic esophagitis over three decades in Olmsted County, Minnesota. Clin Gastroenterol Hepatol 2009;7(10):1055–61.
51. Jensen ET, Kappelman MD, Kim HP, et al. Early life exposures as risk factors for pediatric eosinophilic esophagitis. J Pediatr Gastroenterol Nutr 2013;57(1): 67–71.
52. Greenhawt M, Aceves SS, Spergel JM, et al. The management of eosinophilic esophagitis. J Allergy Clin Immunol Pract 2013;1(4):332–40.
53. Aceves SS. Food allergy testing in eosinophilic esophagitis: what the gastroenterologist needs to know. Clin Gastroenterol Hepatol 2014;12(8):1216–23.
54. Gonsalves N, Yang GY, Doerfler B, et al. Elimination diet effectively treats eosinophilic esophagitis in adults; food reintroduction identifies causative factors. Gastroenterology 2012;142(7):1451–9.
55. Clayton F, Fang JC, Gleich GJ, et al. Eosinophilic esophagitis in adults is associated with IgG4 and not mediated by IgE. Gastroenterology 2014;147(3):602–9.
56. Rothenberg ME. Molecular, genetic, and cellular bases for treating eosinophilic esophagitis. Gastroenterology 2015;148(6):1143–57.
57. Hirano I, Aceves SS. Clinical implications and pathogenesis of esophageal remodeling in eosinophilic esophagitis. Gastroenterol Clin North Am 2014;43(2): 297–316.
58. Aceves SS, Newbury RO, Dohil R, et al. Esophageal remodeling in pediatric eosinophilic esophagitis. J Allergy Clin Immunol 2007;119(1):206–12.
59. Straumann A. Treatment of eosinophilic esophagitis: diet, drugs, or dilation? Gastroenterology 2012;142(7):1409–11.
60. Dellon E. Management of refractory eosinophilic oesophagitis. Nat Rev Gastroenterol Hepatol 2017;14(8):479–90.
61. Schaefer ET, Fitzgerald JF, Molleston JP, et al. Comparison of oral prednisone and topical fluticasone in the treatment of eosinophilic esophagitis: a randomized trial in children. Clin Gastroenterol Hepatol 2008;6(2):165–73.
62. Markowitz JE, Spergel JM, Ruchelli E, et al. Elemental diet is an effective treatment for eosinophilic esophagitis in children and adolescents. Am J Gastroenterol 2003;98(4):777–82.
63. Wolf WA, Jerath MR, Sperry SLW, et al. Dietary elimination therapy is an effective option for adults with eosinophilic esophagitis. Clin Gastroenterol Hepatol 2014; 12(8):1272–9.
64. Arias Á, González-Cervera J, Tenias JM, et al. Efficacy of dietary interventions for inducing histologic remission in patients with eosinophilic esophagitis: a systematic review and meta-analysis. Gastroenterology 2014;146(7):1639–48.
65. Henderson CJ, Abonia JP, King EC, et al. Comparative dietary therapy effectiveness in remission of pediatric eosinophilic esophagitis. J Allergy Clin Immunol 2012;129(6):1570–8.
66. Spergel JM, Brown-Whitehorn TF, Cianferoni A, et al. Identification of causative foods in children with eosinophilic esophagitis treated with an elimination diet. J Allergy Clin Immunol 2012;130(2):461–7.
67. Molina-Infante J, Ferrando-Lamana L, Ripoll C, et al. Esophageal eosinophilic infiltration responds to proton pump inhibition in most adults. Clin Gastroenterol Hepatol 2011;9(2):110–7.
68. Lucendo AJ, Arias Á, Molina-Infante J. Efficacy of proton pump inhibitor drugs for inducing clinical and histologic remission in patients with symptomatic esophageal eosinophilia: a systematic review and meta-analysis. Clin Gastroenterol Hepatol 2016;14(1):13–22.

69. Gutiérrez-Junquera C, Fernández-Fernández S, Cilleruelo ML, et al. High preva-lence of response to proton-pump inhibitor treatment in children with esophageal eosinophilia. J Pediatr Gastroenterol Nutr 2016;62(5):704–10.

70. Molina-Infante J, Rodriguez-Sanchez J, Martinek J, et al. Long-term loss of response in proton pump inhibitor-responsive esophageal eosinophilia is uncom-mon and influenced by CYP2C19 genotype and rhinoconjunctivitis. Am J Gastro-enterol 2015;110(11):1567–75.

71. Chuang MY, Chinnaratha MA, Hancock DG, et al. Topical steroid therapy for the treatment of eosinophilic esophagitis (EOE): a systematic review and meta-anal-ysis. Clin Transl Gastroenterol 2015;6:e82.

72. Cotton CC, Eluri S, Wolf WA, et al. Six-food elimination diet and topical steroids are effective for eosinophilic esophagitis: a meta-regression. Dig Dis Sci 2017; 62(9):2408–20.

73. Konikoff MR, Noel RJ, Blanchard C, et al. A randomized, double-blind, placebo-controlled trial of fluticasone propionate for pediatric eosinophilic esophagitis. Gastroenterology 2006;131(5):1381–91.

74. Lindberg GM, Van Eldik R, Saboorian MH. A case of herpes esophagitis after flu-ticasone propionate for eosinophilic esophagitis. Nat Clin Pract Gastroenterol Hepatol 2008;5(9):527–30.

75. Philpott H, Dougherty M, Reed CC, et al. Systematic review: adrenal insufficiency secondary to swallowed topical corticosteroids in eosinophilic esophagitis. Aliment Pharmacol Ther 2018;47(8):1071–8.

76. Philpott H, Nandurkar S, Royce SG, et al. Allergy tests do not predict food trig-gers in adult patients with eosinophilic oesophagitis. A comprehensive prospec-tive study using five modalities. Aliment Pharmacol Ther 2016;44(3):223–33.

77. Groetch M, Venter C, Skypala I, et al. Dietary therapy and nutrition management of eosinophilic esophagitis: a work group report of the American Academy of Al-lergy, Asthma, and Immunology. J Allergy Clin Immunol Pract 2017;5(2):312–24.

78. Schoepfer AM, Gonsalves N, Bussmann C, et al. Esophageal dilation in eosino-philic esophagitis: effectiveness, safety, and impact on the underlying inflamma-tion. Am J Gastroenterol 2010;105(5):1062–70.

79. Egan JV, Baron TH, Adler DG, et al. Esophageal dilation. Gastrointest Endosc 2006;63(6):755–60.

80. Tabatabaei N, Kang D, Wu T, et al. Tethered confocal endomicroscopy capsule for diagnosis and monitoring of eosinophilic esophagitis. Biomed Opt Express 2014;5(1):197.

81. Friedlander JA, Deboer EM, Soden JS, et al. Unsedated transnasal esophago-scopy for monitoring therapy in pediatric eosinophilic esophagitis. Gastrointest Endosc 2016;83(2):299–306.

82. Katzka DA, Smyrk TC, Alexander JA, et al. Accuracy and safety of the cyto-sponge for assessing histologic activity in eosinophilic esophagitis: a two-center study. Am J Gastroenterol 2017;112(10):1538–44.

83. Furuta GT, Kagalwalla AF, Lee JJ, et al. The oesophageal string test: a novel, mini-mally invasive method measures mucosal inflammation in eosinophilic oesopha-gitis. Gut 2013;62(10):1395–405.

84. Wen T, Stucke EM, Grotjan TM, et al. Molecular diagnosis of eosinophilic esoph-agitis by gene expression profiling. Gastroenterology 2013;145(6):1289–99.

85. Butz BK, Wen T, Gleich GJ, et al. Efficacy, dose reduction, and resistance to high-dose fluticasone in patients with eosinophilic esophagitis. Gastroenterology 2014;147(2):324–33.

86. Dellon ES, Rusin S, Gebhart J, et al. Utility of a noninvasive serum biomarker panel for diagnosis and monitoring of eosinophilic esophagitis: a prospective study. Am J Gastroenterol 2016;2015(6):821–7.
87. Wright B, Ochkur S, Olson N, et al. Normalized serum eosinophil peroxidase levels are inversely correlated with esophageal eosinophilia in eosinophilic esophagitis. Dis Esophagus 2018;31(2). https://doi.org/10.1093/dote/dox139.
88. Miehlke S, Hruz P, Von Arnim U, et al. Two new budesonide formulations are highly efficient for treatment of active eosinophilic esophagitis: results from a randomized, double-blind, double-dummy, placebo-controlled multicenter trial. Gastroenterology 2014;146(5):S-16.
89. Dellon ES, Katzka DA, Collins MH, et al. Budesonide oral suspension improves symptomatic, endoscopic, and histologic parameters compared with placebo in patients with eosinophilic esophagitis. Gastroenterology 2017;152(4):776–86.
90. Cheng E, Zhang X, Wilson KS, et al. JAK-STAT6 pathway inhibitors block eotaxin-3 secretion by epithelial cells and fibroblasts from esophageal eosinophilia patients: promising agents to improve inflammation and prevent fibrosis in EoE. PLoS One 2016;11(6):e0157376.
91. Straumann A, Bussmann C, Perkins M. Treatment of eosinophilic esophagitis with the CRTH2-antagonist OCT000459: a novel therapeutic principle [abstract: 856]. Gastroenterology 2012;142(suppl 1):s-147.
92. Spergel JM, Rothenberg ME, Collins MH, et al. Reslizumab in children and adolescents with eosinophilic esophagitis: results of a double-blind, randomized, placebo-controlled trial. J Allergy Clin Immunol 2012;129(2):456–63.e3.
93. Straumann A, Conus S, Grzonka P, et al. Anti-interleukin-5 antibody treatment (mepolizumab) in active eosinophilic oesophagitis: a randomised, placebo-controlled, double-blind trial. Gut 2010;59(1):21–30.
94. Assa'ad AH, Gupta SK, Collins MH, et al. An antibody against IL-5 reduces numbers of esophageal intraepithelial eosinophils in children with eosinophilic esophagitis. Gastroenterology 2011;141(5):1593–604.
95. Rothenberg M, Wen T, Greenberg A, et al. A randomized, double-blind, placebo controlled trial of a novel recombinant, humanized, anti-interleukin-13 monoclonal antibody (RPC4046) in patients with active eosinophilic esophagitis: results of the HEROES study. United European Gastroenterol J 2016;4(Suppl):OP325.
96. Rothenberg ME, Wen T, Greenberg A, et al. Intravenous anti-IL-13 mAb QAX576 for the treatment of eosinophilic esophagitis. J Allergy Clin Immunol 2015;135(2): 500–7.
97. Hirano I, Dellon E, Hamilton J, et al. Dupilumab efficacy and safety in adult patients with active eosinophilic esophagitis: a randomized double-blind placebo-controlled phase 2 trial. Am J Gastroenterol 2017;112(Suppl1):AB 20 (ACG 2017).
98. Dellon ES, Jones PD, Martin NB, et al. Health-care transition from pediatric to adult-focused gastroenterology in patients with eosinophilic esophagitis. Dis Esophagus 2013;26(1):7–13.
99. Eluri S, Book WM, Kodroff E, et al. Lack of knowledge and low readiness for health care transition in eosinophilic esophagitis and eosinophilic gastroenteritis. J Pediatr Gastroenterol Nutr 2017;65(1):53–7.

The Revolution in Treatment of Hepatitis C

Jordan Mayberry, PA-C, William M. Lee, MD*

KEYWORDS

- Direct-acting antivirals • Sustained viral response • Hepatitis C virus
- Protease inhibitors • Polymerase inhibitors

KEY POINTS

- Hepatitis C infection typically goes unrecognized at onset and develops into a chronic infection that can lead to cirrhosis, liver failure and liver cancer.
- Novel treatments that are safe, without significant side effects and nearly 100% effective became available in the last 5 years.
- Sustained viral response (SVR–no virus detectable 12 weeks after end of treatment) is synonymous with life-long cure.
- SVR patients with cirrhosis require ongoing surveillance for liver cancer.
- Remaining challenges include identifying those who are not aware but have infection and providing treatment for those lacking funding.

INTRODUCTION

Over the course of the last 50 years, hepatitis A, B, C, D, and E have been identified; diagnostic testing developed for all five viruses; and treatments established for the two main chronic forms of viral liver infection, hepatitis B and C. Although viral hepatitis was recognized in the 1950s, it was only 50 years ago, that distinctions were made between the different viruses as transmissible agents, separating parenteral transmission from fecal oral transmission. In the 1960s, hepatitis B was identified via the discovery of the Australia antigen (what is now termed HBsAg)[1] and shortly thereafter, an enterovirus identified in the stool of Army recruits was determined to be the causative agent of hepatitis A.[2] Once serologic testing for hepatitis A and B became available in the 1970s, hepatitis B transmission by blood transfusions was eliminated; hepatitis A was confirmed to be rarely if ever transfusion-related and

Division of Digestive and Liver Diseases, University of Texas Southwestern Medical Center at Dallas, Dallas, TX, USA
* Corresponding author. UT Southwestern Medical Center at Dallas, 5959 Harry Hines Boulevard, Suite 420, Dallas, TX 75390-8887.
E-mail address: William.Lee@utsouthwestern.edu

Med Clin N Am 103 (2019) 43–55
https://doi.org/10.1016/j.mcna.2018.08.007
0025-7125/19/© 2018 Elsevier Inc. All rights reserved.

became readily diagnosable with antibody testing for hepatitis A IgM and IgG antibodies, indicating, respectively, current or past infection. At that point, it was evident that many individuals still became infected after blood transfusions or injection drug use (IDU) with a virus that was not hepatitis A or B. By the 1980s, this virus became known as the non-A, non-B virus.[3] By the end of the decade, imaginative and painstaking molecular cloning studies led to the initial detection of fragments of the non-A, non-B virus, now known as hepatitis C virus (HCV).[4] As with hepatitis B earlier, once HCV was sequenced and antibody testing developed, screening of the blood supply became widespread leading to eradication of virtually all post-transfusion hepatitis.[5] By the early 1990s, hepatitis C was eliminated from the blood supply but not before several million individuals in the United States had become infected, only in part because of transfusion-related infection. HCV is not a novel virus and is a member of the hepacivirus family of RNA flaviviruses, closely related to the yellow fever virus. HCV is found world-wide, and seems to have spread rapidly during the period from the 1960s through the 1980s, resulting in nearly 4 million Americans being afflicted with chronic hepatitis C infection. Tragically, even now, more than 50% of people with hepatitis C are unaware of their infection.

During the 1990s, treatment of hepatitis C with interferon therapy began and produced some (but not many) cures early on, but was associated with significant side effects, including fever, flulike symptoms, and depression. Improvements in interferon therapy included the use of pegylated (long-acting) interferons, and combining interferon dosing with oral ribavirin that doubled efficacy. Thereafter, use of interferon/ribavirin combinations continued for more than 20 years. Further advances in the molecular understanding of this virus moved quickly so that by 2014, 25 years after the virus was identified, remarkably effective treatments quickly became available that far surpassed all prior interferon-based regimens in efficacy, tolerability, and safety. This truly was a revolution that found even hepatologists and infectious disease specialists stunned by the rapid transformation of a hard-to-treat disease to simple, safe and effective treatment that can be offered to anyone.

This review focuses on hepatitis C epidemiology; the clinical impact and consequences; some discussion of past hepatitis C treatments; followed by a review of current recommendations for screening, diagnosis, and treatment of this ubiquitous virus.

EPIDEMIOLOGY

Viral hepatitis is the seventh leading cause of death worldwide.[6] Despite a decline in the incidence of most reportable infections, hepatitis C is still on the increase (**Figs. 1** and **2**). Sadly, after a decline in the incidence of acute hepatitis C in the early 2000s, there is currently a rapid rebound, a 133% increase in acute hepatitis C cases,[7,8] largely caused by the opioid epidemic (**Fig. 3**). Identifying chronic hepatitis C has been a great priority, and is increasingly important now that there is universally effective treatment. In 2012, the US Centers for Disease Control and Prevention issued a statement indicating that hepatitis C screening should target baby boomers[9] born between 1945 and 1965, who are (in 2018) between the ages 53 and 73, based on data collected over decades by the National Health and Nutrition Examination Survey. Previously, physicians were generally advised to ask about prior exposures: transfusions before 1992 and any IDU. However, past or casual IDU is not reliably reported by patients perhaps out of shame or just not recalling an event 20 to 30 years prior. The National Health and Nutrition Examination Survey finding that more than 2 million Americans (1 in 30 baby boomers) have hepatitis C has led to the new advice to screen all patients in the

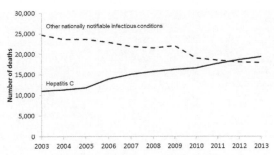

Fig. 1. Deaths related to hepatitis C have been on the increase, whereas death rates for other infectious diseases are declining. (*From* Ly KN, Hughes EM, Jiles RB, et al. Rising mortality associated with hepatitis C virus in the United States, 2003–2013. Clin Infect Dis 2016;62(10):1288; with permission.)

baby boomer cohort, without asking about risk factors. Currently, many electronic medical record systems contain best practice alerts for clinicians to test all patients in this cohort if they have not been previously tested. Some experts believe that all individuals should be screened at some point for hepatitis C because the risk of chronic hepatitis C after initial exposure is high and acute infection often unrecognized.

RISK FACTORS FOR HEPATITIS C

Beyond IDU and transfusions before 1992, sexual contact is a risk factor, largely confined to those with multiple sex partners, other sexually transmitted diseases, and/or high viral loads, which may be observed with combined human immunodeficiency virus (HIV) and HCV infections. Individuals at risk of transmission where treatment will interrupt the transmission cycle include men who have sex with men, active IDUs, incarcerated persons, dialysis patients, and health care workers exposed to blood or blood products. Despite the caution regarding sexual transmission, transmission from one partner to the other is rare for monogamous couples.

NATURAL HISTORY

Most of those who develop hepatitis C viremia go on to chronic infection as indicated in **Fig. 4**, which indicates the fraction of patients in each step along the journey from

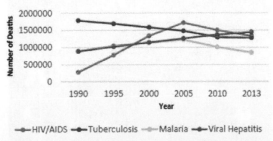

Fig. 2. Estimated deaths worldwide, from viral hepatitis, HIV/AIDS, tuberculosis, and malaria. Other infectious diseases are declining, whereas hepatitis C continues to increase as a cause of death. HIV, human immunodeficiency virus. (*From* IHME. 2016. Global burden of disease study 2013 (GBD 2013) data downloads—full results. http://ghdx.healthdata.org/global-burden-disease-study-2013-gbd-2013-data-downloads-full-results (Accessed March 14, 2016); with permission.)

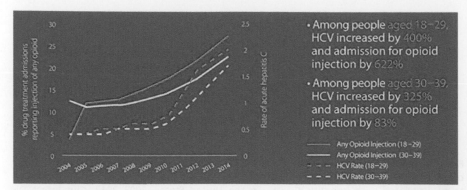

Fig. 3. As the opioid epidemic evolved, cases of acute hepatitis C have increased in parallel; a discouraging finding. (*From* Centers for Disease Control and Prevention (CDC). NCHHSTP Newsroom. Increase in hepatitis C infections linked to worsening opioid crisis. Available at: https://www.cdc.gov/nchhstp/newsroom/2017/hepatitis-c-and-opioid-injection-press-release.html. Accessed May 21, 2018.)

acute to chronic infection and cirrhosis.[9] About 3% of patients with cirrhosis develop liver cancer each year. Overall, only a fraction of patients (perhaps 30% over a lifetime) develop cirrhosis or its sequelae, but this still represents many thousands of patients because of the ubiquity of the disease and an annual death rate of about 50,000 in the United States alone. Risk factors for progression include male gender, length of infection, concomitant alcohol abuse, and nonalcoholic fatty liver disease (NAFLD).[10]

VIROLOGY

This RNA virus includes a single stranded genome of more than 9000 nucleotides (**Fig. 5**), that encodes a single protein that can be cleaved by a protease enzyme to its components. Replication takes place in the hepatocyte cytoplasm; certain details of the virus life cycle are still not fully understood. The targets of the direct-acting antivirals (DAAs) are the components of virus assembly. For example, protease inhibitors bind at

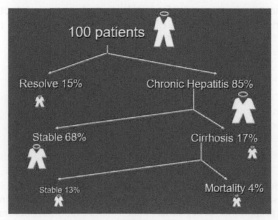

Fig. 4. Outcomes of hepatitis C infection over time. Only 15% are estimated to resolve acute hepatitis C infection, whereas the remainder become chronically infected, leading to cirrhosis and liver cancer in some but not all who remain chronically infected.

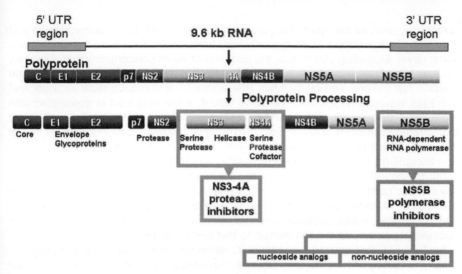

Fig. 5. Schematic of the structure of the hepatitis C virus. (*From* McGovern BH, Abu Dayyeh BK, Chung RT. Avoiding therapeutic pitfalls: the rational use of specifically targeted agents against hepatitis C infection. Hepatology 2008;48(5):1701; with permission.)

the nonstructural (NS) NS3 site to inhibit production of the protease; likewise, the various other NS protein loci have been targeted with nucleoside and nonnucleoside analogues that interfere with replication via halting transcription in the NS5A and NS5B regions.

ACUTE HEPATITIS C

It is estimated that only 10% of acute hepatitis C infections are clinically evident; thus, most are unrecognized and most become chronic. Overall, more acute infections that are symptomatic result in viral clearance (perhaps 50%) than among those that remain without evident hepatitis symptoms.[9] Acute hepatitis C has an incubation period of 1 to 3 weeks, and when clinically apparent yields symptoms of nausea, vomiting, fatigue, and jaundice. Liver enzyme (aspartate aminotransferase and alanine aminotransferase) levels may reach the low 1000 range but seldom are higher than 2000 IU/L, whereas bilirubin levels are rarely higher than 10 to 15 mg/dL.

Antibody to hepatitis C (anti-HCV) develops rapidly but may not be detectable at onset of symptoms. This occasionally results in a missed diagnosis; if clinical hepatitis is present and the initial hepatitis C antibody test is negative, it is prudent to repeat testing a week later. In the early stages of infection, HCV RNA should be detectable, even with a negative antibody test, which may be useful in certain settings. HCV RNA alone indicates viremia even in the absence of hepatitis C antibody, which can occasionally be seen in immunosuppression or advanced HIV infection. Unlike hepatitis A and B, IgM antibody is not meaningful as a test to indicate the acuity of infection. It is difficult to prove the diagnosis of acute hepatitis C unless previously negative anti-HCV data are available for the patient in question. Thus, the diagnosis of acute hepatitis C is based on a recent onset of acute hepatitis with a positive anti-HCV (confirmed with an HCV RNA test) in the absence of known chronic hepatitis C.

CHRONIC HEPATITIS C

For the most part, chronic hepatitis C infection is not associated with discernible clinical effects over the first years of infection. Some patients complain of subjective symptoms, such as low-grade fatigue and malaise. Aspartate aminotransferase and alanine aminotransferase levels typically vary from normal to two- to four-fold elevations, rarely exceeding 200 IU/L in the absence of other concomitant liver diseases, such as NAFLD or alcoholic liver injury. Viral RNA is measured by polymerase chain reaction but the precise viral load has little significance in most clinical settings, and averages around 2 million IU/L. To some extent, a low viral load is associated with more rapid disease resolution during treatment, but is not associated with lower aminotransferase levels or fewer clinical symptoms. Likewise, patients with a high viral load do not seem to progress more rapidly than patients with a low viral load with a few rare exceptions, such as fibrosing cholestatic hepatitis C (discussed later). Some patients complain of fatigue or lack of energy but this is nonspecific and cannot be tied to any specific pattern of disease short of cirrhosis. Thus, patients may remain unaware of illness for decades; screening at annual checkups often is the time when the infection is revealed, either because abnormal aminotransferase levels are detected or because physicians have been alerted to test certain patient groups.

Acute liver failure caused by hepatitis C alone has almost never been reported.[11] When liver failure occurs, this may represent acute hepatitis C superimposed on other liver diseases, such as NAFLD or alcoholic liver disease. Rapid progression to cirrhosis and liver failure with jaundice may rarely occur following intense immunosuppression, and has been termed fibrosing cholestatic hepatitis C.[12] This may occur in the patient with HIV with low CD4 count or occasionally after liver transplantation. With new DAAs readily available, fibrosing cholestatic hepatitis C should become a thing of the past.

Extrahepatic manifestations of hepatitis C are legion and vary greatly affecting nearly every organ system (**Box 1**), from corneal ulcers (very rare) to leukocytoclastic vasculitis involving the lower extremities as a result of cryoglobulinemia. Positive rheumatoid factor is present in 30% or more of patients with chronic hepatitis C and is evidence of the cryoglobulins that can result in glomerular injury and renal failure. In general, resolution of the viral infection results in diminishing cryoglobulin levels but not necessarily full resolution of the cryoglobulin-associated diseases.[13]

Box 1
Partial list of extrahepatic manifestations of hepatitis C

Mixed cryoglobulinemia causing vasculitis, with dermatologic, neuropathic, and renal injury

B-cell lymphomas

Type II diabetes mellitus

Immune thrombocytopenia

Sicca syndrome

Positive rheumatoid factor and other autoantibodies

Hyperglobulinemia

Porphyria cutanea tarda

Lichen planus

Polymyositis

Polyarteritis nodosa

Mooren corneal ulcer

CIRRHOSIS

For decades, hepatitis C has been the most common cause of cirrhosis in the United States, but may soon be displaced by fatty liver disease. Hepatitis C remains the most common indication for liver transplantation in North America. Cirrhosis is defined as the presence of fibrosis and nodule formation and results from ongoing chronic low-grade inflammation and hepatocyte necrosis. As shown in **Fig. 4**, not all HCV patients develop cirrhosis. Some estimates suggest that only 20% to 30% of HCV infections lead to cirrhosis and a smaller percentage of those progress to complications of cirrhosis. Thus, even patients with cirrhosis may elude diagnosis until complications ensue. Whether cirrhosis develops depends on several cofactors. Gender (male less favorable), age (older less favorable), alcohol use, and obesity (fatty liver) all predispose to more rapid cirrhosis progression, which develops roughly 20 years following onset of infection. Liver biopsies may be performed at all stages of disease and are helpful as a prognostic tool. Biopsies are graded for degree of inflammation (0–4) and stage of fibrosis (0–4).

Decompensation is defined as the development of cirrhosis complications: ascites, hepatic encephalopathy, spontaneous bacterial peritonitis, or variceal hemorrhage. The occurrence of any of these complications heralds a significant decrease in life expectancy. The 5-year survival of patients with cirrhosis without complications of nearly 90% falls to approximately 50% 5-year survival once decompensation occurs. Treatment aimed at elimination of the virus results in improvement in aminotransferase levels, decreased inflammation, and essentially no further evolution of the cirrhosis process. Some degree of reversion to earlier stage disease may occur, but once cirrhosis is present it is seldom reversible to any great extent.[14]

PRETREATMENT TESTING

After establishing that the patient has chronic hepatitis C via antibody testing and confirmation with a positive HCV RNA by polymerase chain reaction, further testing is completed to determine the level of fibrosis and the best treatment options (**Fig. 6**). An HCV genotype should be drawn and often is ordered as a reflex test along with the HCV RNA. In addition, it is important to determine the level of fibrosis within the liver, because patients with evidence of cirrhosis often require longer duration of treatment. Fibrosis is graded on liver biopsy from F0 (none) to F4 (cirrhosis). Determining

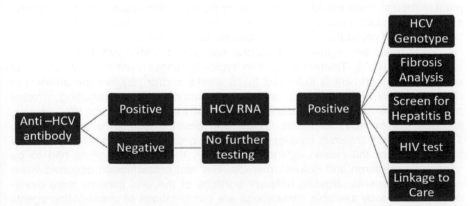

Fig. 6. Simplified schematic diagram of the tests needed before undertaking hepatitis C treatment. Insurers generally require these tests to approve the prescription.

fibrosis stage also allows for planning for care after treatment: patients with cirrhosis and those with bridging fibrosis (F3) also require continued hepatocellular carcinoma screening following eradication of their hepatitis C. There are several modalities for determining fibrosis level including Fibrosure, a series of blood tests that when combined can approximate the histologic fibrosis score; Fibroscan, which measures liver stiffness using sound waves; and ultrasound elastography, another measure of liver stiffness. For hepatitis C, liver biopsy remains the gold standard, but is done less frequently now because of cost, and the more invasive nature of obtaining tissue. Although biopsy is no longer required before treatment, most insurers require and review all of the previously mentioned testing before approval of the treatment prescription. In general, this is accomplished by submitting the required data to a specialty pharmacy that then processes the information and forwards it to the third-party payer for approval, at which point the pharmacy is approved to dispense the medication.

During the initial work-up, all patients with chronic hepatitis C should be screened for hepatitis A and B with testing for anti–hepatitis A virus IgG, HBsAg, anti-HBc, and anti-HBs antibodies. Patients that are not immune to hepatitis A virus and hepatitis B virus (HBV) should be vaccinated against both viruses. Patients with HCV should be screened for HIV because these viruses have similar modes of transmission. Patients with combined HIV and HCV require a multidisciplinary approach, usually beginning with HIV treatment, followed by HCV treatment, once the HIV treatment has been established for 3 to 6 months.

CURRENT TREATMENT OPTIONS FOR HEPATITIS C

The remarkable advances in hepatitis C therapy currently allow for most patients to be treated successfully, regardless of the presence or absence of cirrhosis; hepatitis C genotype; or comorbid conditions, such as HIV or chronic kidney disease.[9] The goal is complete viral eradication, usually determined following HCV RNA testing 12 weeks after the last dose of medication. If there is no virus detectable at this time, the patient is determined to be a sustained viral responder (SVR). SVR confers a >99% likelihood of lifelong viral clearance. It is always advisable to recheck the HCV RNA level at least twice, so that the SVR result at 12 weeks is confirmed by at least one additional measure. There is little evidence that the virus persists in an inactive form or could reactivate with intense immunosuppression. For example, patients who are cured of their hepatitis C before transplantation never relapse post liver transplant. Although there are little data in this area, reinfection caused by re-exposure, such as continued or relapse of IDU, is possible because the hepatitis C antibody is not considered protective but simply indicates past exposure.

Current treatment regimens are all oral and well-tolerated with high SVR rates approaching 100%. Treatment duration typically ranges from 8 to 12 weeks. In some cases, treatment is extended to 16 weeks and/or requires the addition of ribavirin. As with HIV treatment, hepatitis C treatment involves targeting different portions of the virus simultaneously because of the propensity for RNA viruses, such as HIV or HCV, to mutate rapidly and develop resistance to medication. The initial direct antivirals developed were the protease inhibitors telaprevir and boceprevir. For the reason outlined previously, these single agents had to be used with interferon and ribavirin therapy. The real breakthrough occurred when multiple oral agents targeting different portions of the viral genome were developed. All currently available medications are combinations of direct-acting agents from multiple classes (**Table 1**). Choosing a treatment regimen is complex, depending on prior treatment, viral load, presence or absence of cirrhosis, and other

Table 1
Main options for hepatitis C treatment currently available

	Harvoni (Sofosbuvir/ Ledipasvir)	Epclusa (Sofosbuvir/ Velpatasvir)	Zepatier (Elbasvir/ Grazoprevir)	Mavyret (Pibrentasir/ Glecaprevir)	Vosevi (Sofosbuvir/ Velpatasvir/ Voxilaprevir)
Manufacturer	Gilead	Gilead	Merck	Abbvie	Gilead
MOA	NS5B + NS5A	NS5B + NS5A	NS5A + PI	NS5A + PI	NS5B + NS5A + PI
Genotype coverage	1, 4, 5, 6	1, 2, 3, 4, 5, 6	1, 4	1, 2, 3, 4, 5, 6	1, 2, 3, 4, 5, 6
Dosing	Once daily	Once daily	Once daily	Once daily	Once daily

Abbreviation: MOA, mode of action (the part of the virus that the drug inhibits) and protease inhibitor.

factors to determine drug choice and treatment duration. Most clinicians currently follow the remarkably complete and up-to-date treatment recommendations found on the Web site, www.hcvguidelines.org. This site is maintained by the American Association for the Study of Liver Diseases and the Infectious Disease Society of America and is updated regularly, providing unbiased information on the nuances of treating HCV infection. Referring to this one site allows treatment to be uniform, reliable, and precludes the need to memorize complex algorithms, particularly because treatment recommendations do change over time. Most standard regimens are 12 weeks in duration with one combination pill per day (eg, Harvoni). Presence of cirrhosis and high viral load may require 24 weeks of treatment or consideration of 12 weeks of treatment with added ribavirin.

EIGHT-WEEK TREATMENT OPTIONS

Several treatment regimens allow for 8 weeks of treatment based on patient demographics (**Table 2**). Harvoni is used in genotype 1 patients without cirrhosis, treatment naive with pretreatment viral load less than 6 million international units.[15] Mavyret is used for 8 weeks in all genotypes, where patients do not have cirrhosis and are treatment naive. Patients who were previously treated with interferon + Ribavirin + sofosbuvirare are considered treatment naive in this situation.

Table 2
8-week regimens for hepatitis C treatment

	Harvoni (Sofosbuvir/Ledipasvir)	Mavyret (Pibrentasir/ Glecaprevir)
8-wk duration	Yes	Yes
Genotype coverage	1	1, 2, 3, 4, 5, 6
Patient demographics	Noncirrhotic Treatment naive Pretreatment viral load <6 million IU	Noncirrhotic Treatment naive Previously treated with INF + RBV + SOF
Use in renal impairment	No	Yes
Use in decompensated cirrhosis	Yes	No

Abbreviations: INF, interferon; RBV, ribavirin; SOF, sofosbuvir.
Each regimen depends on the patient meeting specified additional criteria.

HEPATITIS B SCREENING

All patients that are being considered for hepatitis C treatment with HCV direct-acting agents should be screened for evidence of current or prior HBV infection before starting therapy. HBV reactivation has been reported in patients taking HCV direct-acting agents who were not on concomitant HBV therapy.[16] Reported cases have included acute liver failure and even death; however, these instances are rare. Recommendations include screening patients with HBsAg and HBcAb. All patients with evidence of HBV/HCV coinfection, such as a positive HBsAg or evidence of serologic resolution (positive HBcAb), should be monitored for HBV reactivation during HCV treatment and following completion of HCV therapy.

Concern has also been raised recently among hepatologists treating hepatitis C patients with DAAs that recurrence of a treated HCC and de novo tumors might be increased in frequency following DAA treatment. Although these outcomes seem unlikely, it is necessary to conduct large prospective trials to confirm or deny these observations.[17]

SPECIAL PATIENT POPULATIONS

Historically, there were several barriers to treatment with interferon-based regimens including comorbidities, such as uncontrolled diabetes, obesity, coinfection with HIV, and race. The direct-acting agents have much fewer barriers. Patients that are coinfected with HIV are no longer considered a special patient population when considering hepatitis C treatment. HIV/HCV coinfected patients are treated for the same duration as monoinfected HCV patients, although attention to avoid medication interactions is necessary. Further information on this topic is available on the HCVguidelines.org Web site.

RENAL DISEASE

Harvoni is not indicated in patients with a glomerular filtration rate less than 30 mL/min/1.73 m^2. Mavyret and Zepatier are used in moderate to severe renal disease including end-stage renal disease. There are no dosage adjustment recommendations for patients with moderate to severe renal disease on Mavyret or Zepatier.

DECOMPENSATED LIVER DISEASE

Treatment regimens containing a protease inhibitor are not indicated for treatment of patients with Childs Pugh B or C liver disease because instances of decompensation have been observed in this setting. Harvoni, because it does not contain a protease inhibitor, is approved for use in patients with decompensated liver disease.

POST-TREATMENT LABORATORY STUDIES AND FOLLOW-UP

SVR is defined as an undetected HCV viral load (by a sensitive assay, <15 IU/mL) 12 weeks after completion of therapy. All patients should have liver fibrosis assessment before starting HCV therapy. Patients demonstrated to have early stage fibrosis (F0-F2) do not require further monitoring (beyond a second RNA test at some point), following eradication of their HCV. Patients that have evidence of advanced fibrosis (F3-F4) should be screened for hepatocellular carcinoma following eradication of their virus. Recommended screening for patients with advanced fibrosis is a liver ultrasound and alpha fetoprotein every 6 months. All patients with known cirrhosis should also be screened for esophageal varices with an esophagogastroduodenoscopy. Survival for patients with inactive cirrhosis after viral eradication should be excellent in the absence of decompensated cirrhosis. Decompensation means symptomatic complications of cirrhosis: esophageal variceal hemorrhage, ascites, hepatic encephalopathy, or spontaneous bacterial peritonitis. Once any episode of decompensation has occurred, the 5-year survival of patients with cirrhosis drops to roughly 50% from the 80% to 90% range. Once patients with cirrhosis develop evidence for decompensation, liver transplant evaluation should be considered.

BARRIERS TO TREATMENT

Despite the availability of several effective and tolerable treatment regimens for hepatitis C, there remain several barriers to treatment of patients with hepatitis C: patient-, physician-, and payer-derived barriers that directly impact access and, indirectly, rates of cure (**Box 2**).[18] Thus, only a small fraction in recent years

---

Box 2
Perceived barriers to HCV treatment

Patient related

- Fear of side effects
- Medication expense
- Laboratory expense
- Low success rate of treatment
- Fear of stigma related to HCV
- Preference for alternative therapy
- Desire to wait for newer therapies
- Difficulty with administration
- Treatment duration
- Patient declines liver biopsy
- Inaccessibility of experienced providers

Government related

- Government restricts treatment
- Insufficient funds allocated to HCV
- Lack of promotion for HCV treatment

Provider related

- Treatment limited to government-mandated centers
- Lack of office infrastructure to treat patients
- Insufficient reimbursement for physicians
- Unable to obtain necessary laboratory studies for treatment
- Limited access to medications or laboratory studies
- Insufficient training for HCV management
- Lack of referral to HCV providers by other physicians
- Lack of proper storage for medications

Payer related
- Insurance plan does not cover treatment
- High out-of-pocket expense for patients
- Restricted insurance coverage for patients with HCV
- Insurance plans do not cover RNA/genotyping
- Excessive paperwork requirements
- Insurance plans limit which physicians treat HCV
- Insurer does not cover serum markers of fibrosis
- Insurance plans do not cover medications for side effects
- Liver biopsy required for treatment

All barriers scored on a 10-point Likert scale, with 0 representing "not a barrier to treatment," 5 representing "somewhat of a barrier to treatment," and 10 representing "large barrier to treatment."

Adapted from McGowan CE, Monis A, Bacon BR, et al. A global view of hepatitis C: physician knowledge, opinions and perceived barriers to care. Hepatology 2013;57(4):1327; with permission.

have been diagnosed and undergone successful treatment (**Fig. 7**). One important barrier continues to be lack of screening for the HCV. Per Centers for Disease Control and Prevention guidelines, all patients born between 1945 and 1965 should have a onetime screening for hepatitis C. Another significant barrier to treatment is insurance coverage for medication. Coverage is plan dependent, and some plans require that patients meet certain guidelines, such as minimum fibrosis scores and a negative routine drug test. Overall, the goal is to treat all patients with active viremia, regardless of disease stage or the presence of symptoms. Treatment of all ensures that we move as a world population closer to eradication of this ubiquitous virus.

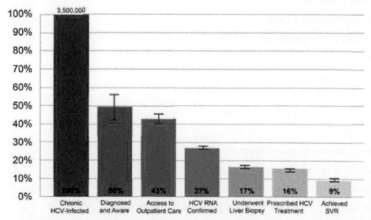

Fig. 7. The treatment cascade for hepatitis C virus infection in the United States. Few, comparatively speaking, receive treatment and are cured of their hepatitis C. (*From* Yehia BR, Schranz AJ, Umscheid CA, et al. The treatment cascade for chronic hepatitis C virus infection in the United States: A systematic review and meta-analysis. PLoS ONE 2014;9(7):e101554; with permission.)

REFERENCES

1. Blumberg BS, Sutnick AI, London WT, et al. Australia antigen and hepatitis. N Engl J Med 1970;283:349–54.
2. Feinstone SM. History of the discovery of hepatitis A virus. Cold Spring Harb Perspect Med 2018. [Epub ahead of print].
3. Seeff L. The history of the "natural history" of hepatitis C (1968-2009). Liver Int 2009;29(Suppl 1):89–99.
4. Houghton M. Discovery of the hepatitis C virus. Liver Int 2009;29(Suppl 1):82–8.
5. Alter HJ, Liang J, Hepatitis C. The end of the beginning or the beginning of the end. Ann Intern Med 2012;156:317–8.
6. Buckley GJ, Strom BL. Eliminating the public health problem of hepatitis B and C in the United States: phase one report. Washington, DC: National Academies of Science, Engineering and Medicine; 2016.
7. Ly KN, Hughes EM, Jiles RB, et al. Rising mortality associated with hepatitis C virus in the United States, 2003-2013. Clin Infect Dis 2016;62:1287–8.
8. Available at: https://www.cdc.gov/nchhstp/newsroom/2017/hepatitis-c-and-opioid-injection-press-release.html. Accessed May 21, 2018.
9. Available at: https://www.cdc.gov/knowmorehepatitis/learnmore.htm. Accessed May 21, 2018.
10. AASLD/IDSA HCV Guidance Panel. Hepatitis C guidance: AASLD-IDSA recommendations for testing, managing and treating adults infected with hepatitis C virus. Hepatology 2015;62:932–54.
11. Thiel AM, Rissland J, Lammert F, et al. Acute liver failure as a rare case of a frequent disease. Z Gastroenterol 2018;56:255–8.
12. Rosenberg PM, Farrell JJ, Abraczinskas DR, et al. Rapidly progressive fibrosing cholestatic hepatitis: hepatitis C virus in HIV coinfection. Am J Gastroenterol 2002;97:478–84.
13. Bunchorntavakul C, Mitrani R, Reddy KR. Advances in HCV and cryoglobulinemic vasculitis in the era of DAAs: are we at the end of the road? J Clin Exp Hepatol 2018;8:81–94.
14. Salmon D, Mondelli MU, Maticic M, et al. The benefits of hepatitis C virus cure: every rose has thorns. J Hepatol 2018;25:320–8.
15. Buggisch P, Zeuzem S. Real-world effectiveness of 8 weeks of treatment with ledipasvir/sofosbuvir in chronic hepatitis C. J Hepatol 2018;68:663–71.
16. Mücke MM, Backus LI, Mücke VT, et al. Hepatitis B virus reactivation during direct-acting antiviral therapy for hepatitis C: a systematic review and meta-analysis. Lancet Gastroenterol Hepatol 2018;3(3):172–80.
17. Calvaruso V, Cabibbo G, Cacciola I, et al. Incidence of hepatocellular carcinoma in patients with HCV-associated cirrhosis treated with direct-acting antiviral agents. Gastroenterology 2018;155(2):411–21.e4.
18. McGowan CE, Monis A, Bacon BR, et al. A global view of hepatitis C: physician knowledge, opinions and perceived barriers to care. Hepatology 2013;57:1325–32.

The Future of Nonalcoholic Fatty Liver Disease Treatment

Khurram Mazhar, MD[a,b],*

KEYWORDS

- Nonalcoholic fatty liver disease • Nonalcoholic steatohepatitis • Obesity
- Metabolic syndrome • Fibrosis

KEY POINTS

- Nonalcoholic fatty liver disease (NAFLD) is a global epidemic and a leading cause of chronic liver disease in the United States.
- The diagnosis of NAFLD rests on obtaining an accurate alcohol intake history, coupled with compatible biochemical, imaging, and histologic features.
- Cirrhosis, cardiovascular morbidity and mortality, as well as liver-related and cancer mortality, are all higher in patients with NAFLD and nonalcoholic steatohepatitis (NASH), the progressive subtype of NAFLD.
- Lifestyle modifications and optimization of metabolic risk factors remains the cornerstone of therapy in NAFLD.
- New therapies for NAFLD and NASH are on the horizon, but appropriate management of obesity and the metabolic syndrome persists as a mainstay of therapy.

INTRODUCTION

Nonalcoholic fatty liver disease (NAFLD) has rapidly become a leading cause of chronic liver disease in the United States. The metabolic comorbidities of central obesity, diabetes mellitus, and dyslipidemia are the most prominent risk factors associated with NAFLD.[1,2]

NAFLD includes a continuum of disease from bland steatosis, which is generally benign, to nonalcoholic steatohepatitis (NASH), which can progress to cirrhosis, liver

---

Disclosure Statement: The author does not have any commercial or financial conflicts of interest.
[a] Department of Internal Medicine, Division of Digestive and Liver Diseases, University of Texas Southwestern Medical Center, North Texas VA Health Care System, Dallas VA Medical Center, 5323 Harry Hines Boulevard, Dallas, TX 75390-9030, USA; [b] Division of Gastroenterology, North Texas VA Health Care System, Dallas VA Medical Center, 111B1, 4500 South Lancaster Road, Dallas, TX 75216, USA
* Division of Gastroenterology, North Texas VA Health Care System, Dallas VA Medical Center, Dallas VA Medical Center, 111B1, 4500 South Lancaster Road, Dallas, TX 75216.
E-mail address: Khurram.Mazhar2@va.gov

failure, and complications of portal hypertension. Hence, it is important to distinguish between these subtypes of NAFLD, as the prognostic and management implications differ. Historically, "cryptogenic" cirrhosis has been defined as the presence of cirrhosis without an obvious etiology. However, studies of patients with cryptogenic cirrhosis show the vast majority of these patients have metabolic syndrome, so may have cirrhosis related to NAFLD.[2–5] As the incidence and prevalence of NAFLD (and its associated complications) are projected to continue rising in the coming years, there has been a renewed push within the hepatology and pharmaceutical communities to develop new therapies to reduce progression to cirrhosis and hepatocellular carcinoma.

To put this rapidly changing landscape of NAFLD therapeutics into greater perspective, in 2013 there were 8 clinical trials for NAFLD treatments registered with ClinicalTrials.gov. By the end of 2015, that number increased to 265, and by April 2016, there were 394 active clinical trials, most of which are being conducted in the United States and Europe.[6] As new medications have allowed cure of hepatitis C, more attention is being focused on the disease that is surpassing hepatitis C as the most common indication for liver transplantation in the United States.

Population-based studies and epidemiologic data vary widely in the estimates of the US population that is affected with NAFLD.[7–9] Between 20% and 40% of the US adult population is affected by NAFLD, and of that group, 4% to 5% have NASH.[7] This translates to roughly 97 million adults with hepatic steatosis and of those, 16 million adults with NASH.

NAFLD affects all genders and ethnicities and occurs in all ages (including children), with prevalence increasing with advancing age.[7–13] Population-based data suggest that NAFLD appears to be most prevalent in Hispanic white, followed by non-Hispanic white individuals, and is least prevalent in non-Hispanic black individuals.[14] Genetic predisposition to NAFLD is an area of study, and several genes have been identified that impair or inhibit lipid mobilization, trafficking, and/or transport in the liver.[15] However, genetic predisposition is only one of the mechanisms contributing to the development of NAFLD and NASH. Other important factors include behavior, lifestyle, metabolic risk factors, and the interaction of the gut microbiome with the immune system.

Identification of patients with the more aggressive subtype of NASH is important, especially if there is underlying hepatic fibrosis. Studies on the natural history of NAFLD and NASH show that patients with hepatic fibrosis are at a higher risk for cirrhosis, liver-related mortality, and all-cause mortality.[16–18] Cardiovascular disease and cancer are among the top causes of death in patients with NAFLD.[16] NAFLD-related hepatocellular carcinoma (NAFLD-HCC) is growing at an incidence rate of 9% per year, as more patients develop NAFLD and NASH.[19,20]

NAFLD has now become the most common cause of chronic liver disease in the United States and the western world, in part due to increasing rates of central obesity and metabolic syndrome. Patients with the more progressive subtype of NASH can progress to cirrhosis, liver failure, HCC, and need liver transplantation. Given the enormous burden of this disease and increased health care utilization due to complications of NAFLD/NASH, early recognition, proactive management, and new treatments are sorely needed.

SYMPTOMS/CLINICAL PRESENTATION

As has been alluded to earlier, NAFLD is the hepatic manifestation of the metabolic syndrome. Risk factors and other associated conditions are noted in **Table 1**. Other

Table 1	
Nonalcoholic fatty liver disease risk factors and associated conditions	
Known Risk Factors	**Suspected Risk Factors**
Obesity	Hypothyroidism
Type 2 diabetes mellitus	Obstructive sleep apnea
Dyslipidemia	Hypogonadism
Metabolic Syndrome	Pancreaticoduodenal resection
	Total parenteral nutrition

lesser-known, but equally important causes of NAFLD can include protein-calorie malnutrition, rapid weight loss, medications, lipodystrophy, dysbetalipoproteinemia, and polycystic ovary syndrome.[4,21,22] Evaluation for these conditions can be considered in the appropriate clinical context.

CLINICAL FEATURES

The vast majority of patients are asymptomatic on diagnosis. There may be nonspecific complaints of fatigue, abdominal fullness, malaise, or right upper quadrant discomfort. Physical examination findings include elevated body mass index (BMI) (patients with BMI >25 are considered to be higher risk), elevated blood pressure, hepatomegaly, and acanthosis nigricans in children and younger adults.[22,23] In patients with advanced hepatic fibrosis or compensated cirrhosis, stigmata of chronic liver disease may be present, but are more commonly absent.

DIAGNOSTIC TESTING, IMAGING, AND ADDITIONAL EVALUATION

One critical aspect of diagnosing NAFLD is to reliably exclude excessive alcohol consumption. This can be challenging because patients may underestimate or overtly deny their true alcohol intake. Corroborating the patient's alcohol consumption history with significant others, family members, and friends can be useful in some situations. Most NAFLD studies and the recently published practice guidance statements from the American Association for the Study of Liver Diseases (AASLD) on the diagnosis and management of NAFLD state that, "ongoing or recent alcohol consumption >21 standard drinks on average per week in men and greater than 14 standard drinks on average per week in women is a reasonable threshold for significant alcohol consumption when evaluating patients with suspected NAFLD."[4,24,25]

It is important to remember that NAFLD is a diagnosis of exclusion. Other causes of chronic liver disease should be ruled out, including viral causes (hepatitis B virus, hepatitis C virus), alcoholic liver disease, autoimmune hepatitis, hereditary hemochromatosis, and Wilson disease (especially in younger patients).[25] A review of the patient's current medications, including over-the-counter and herbal supplements is essential, as some medications and supplements can contribute to chronic liver disease and steatosis. Patient with NAFLD and other contributors to chronic liver disease can progress more quickly to advanced hepatic fibrosis or cirrhosis.

Biochemical Features

With NAFLD, the hepatocellular liver enzymes aspartate aminotransferase (AST) and alanine aminotransferase (ALT) can be mildly elevated and fluctuate over time. These elevations are usually 2 to 5 times the upper limit of normal. Cholestatic elevations in alkaline phosphatase, gamma glutamyltransferase, and bilirubin may also occur in conjunction with elevated aminotransferases, but rarely are these increased in an isolated manner without a concomitant elevation in AST and ALT. Hyperbilirubinemia, hypoalbuminemia, and coagulopathy are indicative of advanced liver disease and cirrhosis. As liver enzyme levels in NAFLD will fluctuate, patients with normal liver enzymes can still have hepatic steatosis. In fact, 78% of patients with NAFLD can have normal aminotransferase levels at any one time.[26] Therefore, a single "snapshot in time" check of liver transaminases is not an adequate screening mechanism for NAFLD. Serial measurement of liver enzyme levels over several months, in conjunction with a compatible history, imaging, histology, and the exclusion of competing etiologies for chronic liver disease, are important for diagnosis.

During the biochemical workup of patients with abnormal liver tests and suspected NAFLD, other tests, such as serum iron tests and autoantibodies, may be abnormal. This can lead to confusion regarding the presence of a true iron overload state or autoimmune condition. Further testing for hereditary hemochromatosis may be considered. It should be noted that ferritin levels are usually only mildly to modestly elevated in NAFLD and are likely a reflection of chronic hepatitis with an unclear impact on disease progression.[27,28] Autoantibody titers (the most common being antinuclear antibody) can be weakly positive (typically <1:40 titer) in NAFLD. Mildly elevated autoantibody titers are considered clinically insignificant and do not have an impact on more advanced disease or atypical histologic features.[29]

Imaging Features

Radiological imaging techniques are frequently used to help in the diagnosis of NAFLD, as clinical and laboratory tests are nonspecific. Ultrasonography, computed tomography (CT), and MRI can all be used to noninvasively diagnose hepatic steatosis. On ultrasonography, hepatic steatosis will frequently cause increased echogenicity of the hepatic parenchyma compared with the spleen or kidney.[30,31] The ability of ultrasonography to detect steatosis can be highly sensitive and specific (upwards of 95%); however, obesity decreases the sensitivity and specificity of ultrasonography, due to the impaired ability of the ultrasound beam to penetrate the subcutaneous and intraabdominal adipose tissue.[31] Although ultrasonography is sensitive for detection of NAFLD, hepatic steatosis can still be present, even with a normal ultrasound.

CT and MRI also can reliably detect hepatic steatosis. Noncontrast CT images will show fatty infiltration of the liver with low attenuation and the liver will appear darker than the spleen. The sensitivity of CT to detect hepatic steatosis is comparable to ultrasonography, approximately 93%. MRI and its various iterations (ie, MR spectroscopy) are also highly sensitive and offer quantitation of the volume of liver fat (>5% liver fat on MR spectroscopy indicates steatosis).[32] Limited availability, cost, and the ability to use less expensive imaging modalities make MRI an impractical method to diagnose hepatic steatosis. At this time, none of the available imaging techniques can differentiate between simple steatosis and NASH.[30]

Histologic Features

NAFL and NASH can be reliably differentiated only by liver biopsy. Clinical history, laboratory data, and imaging studies are unpredictable in determining whether the patient has a more benign or potentially aggressive form of the disease. Moreover, NAFL/NASH can be indistinguishable from liver damage that results from alcoholic liver disease.

Histologically, NAFL is defined as the presence of ≥5% of the available hepatic parenchyma to be infiltrated by fat. Steatosis is predominately macrovesicular in nature and the parenchyma is devoid of significant fibrosis and/or a mixed inflammatory cell infiltrate. By contrast, histologic NASH will have ≥5% hepatic steatosis, coupled with evidence of hepatocellular injury. This injury is characterized by a mixed inflammatory cell infiltrate of neutrophils and lymphocytes, hepatocyte ballooning/ballooning degeneration, and Mallory hyaline. Fibrosis may be present.[33] If present, the collagen is uniquely laid down in a pericellular distribution around the central vein and perisinusoidally around the hepatocytes in zone 3, known as "chicken-wire fibrosis." Other forms of liver disease will demonstrate fibrosis predominately in a portal distribution and expand out to connect "bridges" of fibrosis with adjacent portal tracts.[33–35]

Although liver biopsy is still considered the gold standard for diagnosis and staging of NAFLD and NASH, it is resource-intensive, costly, requires expert interpretation, runs the risk of sampling error, and has a risk for complications. For these reasons, there has been significant interest in the development of alternative assessments that do not involve the need for a biopsy to better assess steatohepatitis and advanced fibrosis in NAFLD.

Noninvasive Assessment of Steatohepatitis and Advanced Fibrosis in Nonalcoholic Fatty Liver Disease

Features of the metabolic syndrome, such as insulin resistance, diabetes mellitus, dyslipidemia, hypertension, and central adiposity, are strong predictors of progressive and more advanced disease. As patients accumulate components of the metabolic syndrome, the risk of NAFLD increases, and patients with NAFLD and multiple risk factors are at a higher risk of adverse outcomes.[36–38] Several NASH-specific circulating biomarkers, such as cytokeratin 18, and other serum proteins related to NASH, are being investigated, but are currently unavailable for routine clinical use.[39]

Patients with existing hepatic fibrosis need to be identified and managed, as unchecked inflammation can hasten the development of advanced fibrosis and cirrhosis. There are several noninvasive tools that can serve as clinical decision aids to predict advanced fibrosis.[40] The NAFLD fibrosis score (NFS) is composed of 6 clinical data points, including the presence/absence of impaired fasting glucose or diabetes, age, BMI, platelet count, albumin, and AST/ALT ratio.[41] A meta-analysis of 13 studies with more than 3000 patients showed that the NFS had an 85% probability of accurately predicting advanced fibrosis.[42] The Fibrosis-4 index is composed of age, AST, ALT, and platelet count and offers dual cutoffs to predict minimal and more advanced fibrosis.[40] The AST-to-platelet ratio index is not sensitive enough to rule out significantly advanced liver disease, but is generally used in combination with other indices to better assess fibrosis status.

Vibration-controlled transient elastography (VCTE, alternatively known as FibroScan) was recently approved by the US Food and Drug Administration (FDA) to measure liver stiffness, and thus fibrosis, in various liver diseases. This technique is a noninvasive way to quickly determine the degree of hepatic fibrosis in a safe, reliable, and effective manner.[43–45] This technique uses a specialized ultrasound transducer, and fibrosis is measured by determining the velocity of returning pulsed ultrasound waves within the liver back to the transducer. Values are reported in kilopascals (kPa); higher values translate to greater liver stiffness, greater shear wave velocities, and higher degrees of fibrosis.[45] VCTE also correlates well with predicting the risk of hepatic decompensation and complications of increased portal pressure. VCTE testing is limited in obese patients, especially BMI greater than 40, with a test failure rate of 88%.[45] Additionally, acute or chronic inflammation, volume overload, cardiac congestion, cholestasis, excessive alcohol use, nonfasting states, and operator inexperience can all influence the liver stiffness measurement.[45] To obtain an accurate test result, patients should fast for at least 3 hours before their examination, not be actively drinking alcohol, be in a euvolemic state, and have a BMI less than 40. An algorithm for evaluation is shown in **Fig. 1**.

MANAGEMENT AND TREATMENT

At this time, there are no published studies addressing the primary prevention of NAFLD. Therefore, because the vast majority of patients with NAFLD already have the associated metabolic comorbidities, appropriate weight control measures, along with aggressive treatment of insulin resistance, diabetes mellitus, and hyperlipidemia are paramount in arresting progression to chronic hepatitis and fibrosis.[46] Nonpharmacologic treatments are effective in all patients with NAFLD at any stage. Pharmacologic interventions should generally be restricted to those patients with biopsy-proven NASH and fibrosis (**Table 2**).

Lifestyle Intervention

Dietary modifications, exercise, and structured weight loss have all been advocated as effective long-term management strategies for patients with NAFLD. Weight loss of at least 3% to 5% has been shown to improve hepatic steatosis in randomized controlled trials, and also can stabilize or normalize ALT levels in patients with NASH.[47] Larger weight loss goals of 7% to 10% have been shown to produce histologic improvements in NASH, including fibrosis.[48] A recent study of 261 patients who underwent preintervention and postintervention liver biopsies showed a direct correlation between weight loss and histopathologic improvements. In fact, patients who achieved greater weight loss showed significant improvements in all features of NASH, including fibrosis. Over the course of this 12-month prospective trial, 94% of the patients who showed at least 5% weight reduction stabilized or improved their postintervention fibrosis scores; however, only 50% of the patients in this trial were able to achieve at least 7% weight loss at 12 months.[49]

Hypocaloric dietary modifications over a sustained period can improve hepatic steatosis. The specific macronutrient composition needed to obtain durable improvements in histopathology is unclear, but data do support a calorie reduction of approximately 750 to 1000 kcal/d to improve hepatic steatosis.[50]

NAFLD also may be improved by physical activity. Exercise alone can potentially prevent or reduce hepatic steatosis; however, the type, intensity, and duration of exercise needed to attain these benefits is unknown.[51,52] Goals of 150 to 200 min/wk or an increase of 60 min/wk of physical activity from a previous lower baseline can

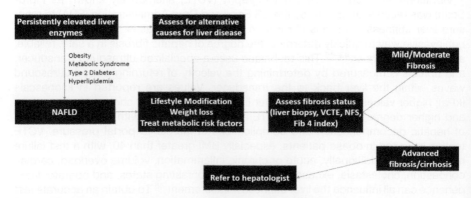

Fig. 1. Algorithm for the management of NAFLD. Fib 4, fibrosis 4.

Table 2
Current therapeutic options in nonalcoholic fatty liver disease

Lifestyle Interventions	Pharmacologic Interventions	Surgical Interventions
Weight Loss 5%–10%	Pioglitazone	Bariatric surgery
Dietary calorie reduction 750–1000 kcal/d	Vitamin E	
Aerobic exercise	Liraglutide	
	Statins	

reduce aminotransferases, independent of weight loss; however, its effects on liver histopathology remain unclear.

Pharmacologic Interventions

Insulin-sensitizing agents

Insulin resistance and diabetes are associated with NAFLD, NASH, and NASH-related fibrosis. Drugs targeting the pathophysiology of insulin resistance are therefore an attractive option independent of lifestyle modifications. Several studies have looked at metformin and its effect on liver histopathology in patients with NAFLD and NASH. Although demonstrating improvements in serum enzyme levels and insulin resistance, a benefit on liver histology is lacking.[53] Therefore, metformin is not considered to be a treatment option for NASH.

The thiazolidinediones are ligands for the peroxisome proliferator-activated receptor (PPAR)-gamma nuclear transcription factor and have effects on glucose and lipid metabolism, as well as insulin sensitization.[54,55] In patients with NASH, rosiglitazone showed improvements in hepatic steatosis, but not fibrosis.[56] At this time, rosiglitazone is rarely used in clinical practice due to increased cardiac events leading to an FDA black box warning.

Pioglitazone has proven to be effective in patients with and without type 2 diabetes and NASH. In a study of 55 patients with biopsy-proven NASH and prediabetes/type 2 diabetes, 45 mg of pioglitazone daily improved insulin sensitivity, serum aminotransferases, and histologic steatosis and inflammation, with a trend toward improvement in fibrosis.[57] In another study of 101 patients with biopsy-proven NASH and early diabetes, 58% of those randomized to pioglitazone 45 mg/d and a hypocaloric diet achieved improvements in histologic parameters and fibrosis, compared with 21% for placebo.[58] The effectiveness of pioglitazone has also been shown in the PIVENS (Pioglitazone vs Vitamin E vs Placebo for the Treatment of Nondiabetic Patients with Nonalcoholic Steatohepatitis) trial. In this study, 34% of patients randomized to 30 mg/d of pioglitazone showed histologic improvement compared with 19% who improved with placebo.[59] The main drawback with pioglitazone treatment, however, is weight gain, theorized to be due to increased triglyceride synthesis and/or improved adipose insulin sensitivity. This limits the clinical use of pioglitazone in routine practice.[58,59]

The glucagon-like peptide-1 (GLP-1) agonist liraglutide is currently in clinical trials for NAFLD and NASH. This GLP-1 agonist reduces appetite, increases insulin sensitivity, increases the transcription of PPAR-gamma, decreases glucose output, and decreases hepatic steatosis.[60]

Vitamin E

Vitamin E is an antioxidant that has been studied as a treatment option for NASH. Oxidative stress is a potential cause of hepatocellular injury and fibrosis progression in NASH. There are multiple studies of vitamin E in NASH, but these studies are heterogeneous with differences in patient eligibility, variable dosing, and limited histologic outcome data. In the PIVENS trial, patients in the vitamin E arm received 800 IU per day, with 43% achieving the primary endpoint of histologic improvement, compared with 19% in the placebo group.[59] Despite its potential effectiveness, there are several unanswered issues related to treating patients with NASH with vitamin E. In the PIVENS trial, 57% of patients did not respond to vitamin E, for unclear reasons. Its efficacy is unproven in patients with diabetes, and the use of liver enzymes as a surrogate marker for improvement (as was used in the PIVENS study) cannot be used to predict disease activity in clinical practice. There are also potential risks associated with long-term use of vitamin E. One meta-analysis concluded that vitamin E at dosages greater than 800 IU per day increased all-cause mortality, although this has not been seen in all studies of vitamin E.[61] Another study showed that vitamin E dosed at 400 IU per day was associated with a modest increase in risk of prostate cancer.[62] The AASLD guidance on vitamin E states that its use can be considered in those patients with biopsy-proven NASH who are not diabetic, with the risks and benefits of the therapy extensively discussed before its initiation.[1,4]

Lipid-lowering medications
Treatment of NASH with HMG-CoA reductase inhibitors (statins) has shown inconsistent results, with some studies showing biochemical improvements and others showing varying effects on histology. However, given the strong association between NAFLD and cardiovascular morbidity and mortality, the use of statins and/or other lipid-lowering medications is advocated for aggressive modification of dyslipidemia.[63] It is important to note that patients with NAFLD and/or NASH are not at a higher risk of hepatotoxicity from statins. Several studies have concluded that statin-induced hepatotoxicity is not any higher in patients with chronic liver disease.[64] Their use should not be avoided in patients with liver disease in daily clinical practice.

Omega-3 fatty acids (fish oil) can be used to treat hypertriglyceridemia in patients with NAFLD,[65] but are not specifically recommended as a primary treatment option for NAFLD.

Miscellaneous agents
Other medications have been studied to assess improvement of NASH and NAFLD. Ursodeoxycholic acid has no histologic benefit in patients with NASH; therefore, it is not a recommended treatment of NAFLD or NASH.[66] Pentoxifylline, a tumor necrosis factor (TNF)-alpha inhibitor, has shown promising results in small studies, with improvements in liver enzymes and insulin resistance. Its effect on histology is less clear, and further studies are needed to determine benefit.[67] Two agents are currently in phase III clinical trials that show promising results. Obeticholic acid, recently FDA-approved for treatment of primary biliary cholangitis, is a Farnesoid-X receptor agonist that has shown improvements in steatohepatitis and fibrosis over 72 weeks in a large, phase II clinical trial.[68] Elafibranor, a dual PPAR-alpha/gamma agonist, has shown improvements in histologic NASH parameters, including stabilization of fibrosis in a recent phase II trial.[69] Several other agents are in early-phase trials at this time, including medications that affect bile and lipid metabolism, incretin mimetics, phosphodiesterase inhibition, TNF modulation, and antifibrotics.

Surgical Intervention

Bariatric surgery improves comorbid diseases in most patients, as well as improving cardiovascular and malignancy-related morbidity and mortality, 2 of the leading causes of death in patients with NAFLD. Although no clinical trials have specifically been performed to evaluate the effect of bariatric surgery on NASH, some studies have shown improvement in the metabolic syndrome, resolution of hepatic steatosis, improvement in liver histology, and resolution of NASH up to 1 and 5 years after bariatric surgery.[70] The safety and efficacy of bariatric surgery in patients with NASH cirrhosis is not firmly established. A recent study did show that compared with patients without cirrhosis (0.3%), mortality after bariatric surgery was minimally higher in those with compensated cirrhosis (0.9%) and much higher in decompensated cirrhosis (16.3%).[71] Therefore, in those patients with compensated NASH cirrhosis, management should be coordinated with an experienced bariatric surgery center.

SUMMARY

NAFLD is a leading cause of chronic liver disease in the United States and the western world. The use of clinical prediction tools and VCTE can help risk stratify patients more effectively and target therapeutic interventions to those patients at a high risk for developing advanced fibrosis and cirrhosis. Although emerging therapeutics are on the horizon, there are currently no FDA-approved therapies for NAFLD and NASH. Although insulin sensitizers, vitamin E, statins, and bariatric surgery can all be used in a multipronged approach, lifestyle modifications, and optimization of metabolic risk factors remain a cornerstone for treatment.

REFERENCES

1. Chalasani N, Younossi Z, Lavine JE, et al. The diagnosis and management of non-alcoholic fatty liver disease: practice guideline by the American Association for the Study of Liver Diseases, American College of Gastroenterology, and the American Gastroenterological Association. Hepatology 2012;55:2005–23.
2. Rinella ME, Sanyal AJ. Management of NAFLD: a stage-based approach. Nat Rev Gastroenterol Hepatol 2016;13:196–205.
3. Collantes R, Ong JP, Younossi ZM. Nonalcoholic fatty liver disease and the epidemic of obesity. Cleve Clin J Med 2004;71:657–64.
4. Chalasani N, Younossi Z, Lavine JE, et al. The diagnosis and management of nonalcoholic fatty liver disease: practice guidance from the American Association for the Study of Liver Diseases. Hepatology 2018;67:328–57.
5. Adams LA, Lymp JF, St Sauver J, et al. The natural history of nonalcoholic fatty liver disease: a population-based cohort study. Gastroenterology 2005;129: 113–21.
6. Website: ClinicalTrials.gov. Available at: https://clinicaltrials.gov/ct2/home. Accessed February 12, 2018.
7. Clark JM, Brancati FL, Diehl AM. The prevalence and etiology of elevated aminotransferase levels in the United States. Am J Gastroenterol 2003;98:960–70.
8. McCullough AJ. The epidemiology and risk factors of NASH. In: Farrell GC, George J, Hall P, et al, editors. Fatty liver disease: NASH and related disorders. Oxford (England): Blackwood Publishing; 2005. p. 23–37.
9. Chang Y, Jung HS, Cho J, et al. Metabolically healthy obesity and the development of nonalcoholic fatty liver disease. Am J Gastroenterol 2016;111:1133–40.
10. Bialek SR, Redd JT, Lynch A, et al. Chronic liver disease among two American Indian patient populations in the southwestern United States, 2000-2003. J Clin Gastroenterol 2008;42:949–54.

11. Fattahi MR, Niknam R, Safarpour A, et al. The prevalence of metabolic syndrome in non-alcoholic fatty liver disease; a population-based study. Middle East J Dig Dis 2016;8:131–7.

12. Koehler EM, Schouten JN, Hansen BE, et al. Prevalence an risk factors of nonalcoholic fatty liver disease in the elderly: results from the Rotterdam study. J Hepatol 2012;57:1305–11.

13. Kangasky N, Levy S, Keter D, et al. Non-alcoholic fatty liver disease–a common and benign finding in octogenarian patients. Liver Int 2004;24:588–94.

14. Masuoka HC, Chalasani N. Nonalcoholic fatty liver disease: an emerging threat to obese and diabetic individuals. Ann N Y Acad Sci 2013;1281:106–22.

15. Dongiovanni P, Anstee QM, Valenti L. Genetic predisposition in NAFLD and NASH: impact on severity of liver disease and response to treatment. Curr Pharm Des 2013;19:5219–38.

16. Younossi Z, Henry L. Contribution of alcoholic and nonalcoholic fatty liver disease to the burden of liver-related morbidity and mortality. Gastroenterology 2016;150: 1778–85.

17. Sayiner M, Koenig A, Henry L, et al. Epidemiology of nonalcoholic fatty liver disease and nonalcoholic steatohepatitis in the United States and the rest of the world. Clin Liver Dis 2016;20:205–14.

18. Sayiner M, Otgonsuren M, Cable R, et al. Variables associated with inpatient and outpatient resource utilization among Medicare beneficiaries with nonalcoholic fatty liver disease with or without cirrhosis. J Clin Gastroenterol 2017;51:254–60.

19. Mohamed B, Shah V, Onyshchenko M, et al. Characterization of hepatocellular carcinoma (HCC) in non-alcoholic fatty liver disease (NAFLD) patients without cirrhosis. Hepatol Int 2016;10:632–9.

20. Younossi ZM, Otgonsuren M, Henry L, et al. Association of nonalcoholic fatty liver disease (NAFLD) with hepatocellular carcinoma (HCC) in the United States from 2004 to 2009. Hepatology 2015;62:1723–30.

21. Angulo P. Nonalcoholic fatty liver disease. In: Talley NJ, Locke GR 3rd, Saito YA, editors. GI epidemiology. Malden (MA): Blackwell Publishing; 2007. p. 883–9.

22. Moscatiello S, Manini R, Marchesini G. Diabetes and liver disease: an ominous association. Nutr Metab Cardiovasc Dis 2007;17:63–70.

23. Matteoni CA, Younossi ZM, Gramlich T, et al. Nonalcoholic fatty liver disease: a spectrum of clinical and pathological severity. Gastroenterology 1999;116: 1413–9.

24. Sanyal AJ, Brunt EM, Kleiner DE, et al. Endpoints and clinical trial design for nonalcoholic steatohepatitis. Hepatology 2011;54:344–53.

25. Liangpunsakul S, Chalasani N. What should we recommend to our patients with NAFLD regarding alcohol use? Am J Gastroenterol 2012;107:976–8.

26. Ekstedt M, Frazen LE, Mathiesen UL, et al. Long-term follow-up of patients with NAFLD and elevated liver enzymes. Hepatology 2006;44:865–73.

27. Kowdley KV, Belt P, Wilson LA, et al. Serum ferritin is an independent predictor of histologic severity and advanced fibrosis in patients with nonalcoholic fatty liver disease. Hepatology 2012;55:77–85.

28. Valenti L, Fracanzani AL, Bugianesi E, et al. HFE genotype, parenchymal iron accumulation, and liver fibrosis in patients with nonalcoholic fatty liver disease. Gastroenterology 2010;138:905–12.

29. Vuppalanchi R, Gould RJ, Wilson LA, et al. Clinical significance of serum autoantibodies in patients with NAFLD: results from the nonalcoholic steatohepatitis clinical research network. Hepatol Int 2012;6:379–85.

30. Saadeh S, Younossi ZM, Remer EM, et al. The utility of radiological imaging in nonalcoholic fatty liver disease. Gastroenterology 2002;123:745–50.
31. Mottin CC, Moretto M, Padoin AV, et al. The role of ultrasound in the diagnosis of hepatic steatosis in morbidly obese patients. Obes Surg 2004;14:635–7.
32. Reeder SB, Cruite I, Hamilton G, et al. Quantitative assessment of liver fat with magnetic resonance imaging and spectroscopy. J Magn Reson Imaging 2011; 34:spcone.
33. Kleiner DE, Brunt EM, Van Natta M, et al, Nonalcoholic Steatohepatitis Clinical Research Network. Design and validation of a histological scoring system for nonalcoholic fatty liver disease. Hepatology 2005;41:1313–21.
34. Bondini S, Kleiner DE, Goodman ZD, et al. Pathologic assessment of non-alcoholic fatty liver disease. Clin Liver Dis 2007;11:17–23.
35. Kleiner DE, Brunt EM. Nonalcoholic fatty liver disease: pathologic patterns and biopsy evaluation in clinical research. Semin Liver Dis 2012;32:3–13.
36. Kang H, Greenson JK, Omo JT, et al. Metabolic syndrome is associated with greater histologic severity, higher carbohydrate, and lower fat diet in patients with NAFLD. Am J Gastroenterol 2006;101:2247–53.
37. Ryan MC, Wilson AM, Slavin J, et al. Associations between liver histology and severity of the metabolic syndrome in subjects with nonalcoholic fatty liver disease. Diabetes Care 2005;28:1222–4.
38. Byrne CD, Targher G. NAFLD: a multisystem disease. J Hepatol 2015;62(1 Suppl):S47–64.
39. Cusi K, Chang Z, Harrison S, et al. Limited value of plasma cytokeratin-18 as a biomarker for NASH and fibrosis in patients with non-alcoholic fatty liver disease. J Hepatol 2014;44:854–62.
40. Kaswala DH, Lai M, Afdhal NH. Fibrosis assessment in nonalcoholic fatty liver disease (NAFLD) in 2016. Dig Dis Sci 2016;61:1356–64.
41. Angulo P, Hui JM, Marchesini G, et al. The NAFLD fibrosis score: a noninvasive system that identifies liver fibrosis in patients with NAFLD. Hepatology 2007;45: 846–54.
42. Musso G, Gambino R, Cassader M, et al. Meta-analysis: natural history of non-alcoholic fatty liver disease (NAFLD) and diagnostic accuracy of non-invasive tests for liver disease severity. Ann Med 2011;43:617–49.
43. Tapper EB, Challies T, Nasser I, et al. The performance of vibration controlled transient elastography in a US cohort of patients with nonalcoholic fatty liver disease. Am J Gastroenterol 2016;111:677–84.
44. Vuppalanchi R, Siddiqui MS, Hallinan EK, et al. Transient elastography is feasible with high success rate for evaluation of non-alcoholic fatty liver disease (NAFLD) in a multicenter setting. Hepatology 2015;62:1290A.
45. Tapper EB, Castera L, Afdhal NH. Fibroscan (vibration-controlled transient elastography): where does it stand in the United States practice. Clin Gastroenterol Hepatol 2015;13:27–36.
46. Kadayifci A, Merriman R, Bass N. Medical treatment of non-alcoholic steatohepatitis. Clin Liver Dis 2007;11:119–40.
47. Promrat K, Kleiner DE, Niemeier HM, et al. Randomized control trial testing the effects of weight loss on nonalcoholic steatohepatitis. Hepatology 2010;51: 121–9.
48. Musso G, Cassader M, Rosina F, et al. Impact of current treatments on liver disease, glucose metabolism and cardiovascular risk in non-alcoholic fatty liver disease (NAFLD): a systematic review and meta-analysis of randomized trials. Diabetologia 2012;55:885–904.

49. Vilar-Gomez E, Martinez-Perez Y, Calzadilla-Bertot L, et al. Weight loss through lifestyle modification significantly reduces features of nonalcoholic steatohepatitis. Gastroenterology 2015;149:367–78.

50. Kirk E, Reeds DN, Finck BN, et al. Dietary fat and carbohydrates differentially alter insulin sensitivity during caloric restriction. Gastroenterology 2009;136:1552–60.

51. Kistler KD, Brunt EM, Clark JM, et al. Physical activity recommendations, exercise intensity, and histological severity of nonalcoholic fatty liver disease. Am J Gastroenterol 2011;106:460–8.

52. St George A, Bauman A, Johnston A, et al. Independent effects of physical activity in patients with nonalcoholic fatty liver disease. Hepatology 2009;50:68–76.

53. Li Y, Liu L, Wang B, et al. Metformin in nonalcoholic fatty liver disease: a systematic review and meta-analysis. Biomed Rep 2013;1:57–64.

54. Yki-Jarvinen H. Thiazolidinediones. N Engl J Med 2004;351:1106–18.

55. Soccio RE, Chen ER, Lazar MA. Thiazolidinediones and the promise of insulin sensitization in type 2 diabetes. Cell Metab 2014;20:573–91.

56. Ratziu V, Charlotte F, Bernhardt C, et al. Long-term efficacy of rosiglitazone in nonalcoholic steatohepatitis: results of the fatty liver improvement by rosiglitazone therapy (FLIRT 2) extension trial. Hepatology 2010;51:445–53.

57. Belfort R, Harrison SA, Brown K, et al. A placebo-controlled trial of pioglitazone in subjects with nonalcoholic steatohepatitis. N Engl J Med 2006;355:2297–307.

58. Cusi K, Orsak B, Bril F, et al. Long-term pioglitazone treatment for patients with nonalcoholic steatohepatitis and prediabetes or type 2 diabetes mellitus: a randomized trial. Ann Intern Med 2016;165:305–15.

59. Sanyal AJ, Chalasani N, Kowdley KV, et al. Pioglitazone, vitamin E, or placebo for non-alcoholic steatohepatitis. N Engl J Med 2010;362:1675–85.

60. Armstrong MJ, Gaunt P, Aithal GP, et al. Liraglutide safety and efficacy in patients with non-alcoholic steatohepatitis (LEAN): a multicenter, double-blind, randomized, placebo-controlled phase 2 study. Lancet 2016;387:679–90.

61. Miller ER, Pastor-Barriuso R, Dalal D, et al. Meta-analysis: high-dosage vitamin E supplementation may increase all-cause mortality. Ann Intern Med 2005;142:37–46.

62. Klein EA, Thompson IM, Tangen CM, et al. Vitamin E and the risk of prostate cancer: the selenium and vitamin E cancer prevention trial (SELECT). JAMA 2011;306:1549–56.

63. Hyogo H, Tazuma S, Arihiro K, et al. Efficacy of atorvastatin for the treatment of nonalcoholic steatohepatitis with dyslipidemia. Metabolism 2008;57:1711–8.

64. Chalasani N, Aljadhey H, Kesterson J, et al. Patients with elevated liver enzymes are not at higher risk for statin hepatotoxicity. Gastroenterology 2004;126:1287–92.

65. Masterton GS, Plevris JN, Hayes PC. Review article: omega-3 fatty acids—a promising novel therapy for non-alcoholic fatty liver disease. Aliment Pharmacol Ther 2010;31:679–92.

66. Lindor KD, Kowdley KV, Heathcote EJ, et al. Ursodeoxycholic acid for treatment of nonalcoholic steatohepatitis: results of a randomized trial. Hepatology 2004;39:770–8.

67. Satapathy SK, Garg S, Chauhan R, et al. Beneficial effects of tumor necrosis factor-alpha inhibition by pentoxifylline on clinical, biochemical, and metabolic parameters of patients with nonalcoholic steatohepatitis. Am J Gastroenterol 2004;99:1946–52.

68. Neuschwander-Tetri BA, Loomba R, Sanyal AJ, et al. Farsenoid X nuclear receptor ligand obeticholic acid for non-cirrhotic, non-alcoholic steatohepatitis (FLINT): a mulitcentre, randomized, placebo-controlled trial. Lancet 2015;385:956–65.
69. Ratziu V, Harrison SA, Francque S, et al. Elafibranor, an agonist of the peroxisome proliferator-activated receptor-alpha and gamma, induces resolution of nonalcoholic steatohepatitis without fibrosis worsening. Gastroenterology 2016;150: 1147–59.
70. Mathurin P, Hollebecque A, Arnalsteen L, et al. Prospective study of the long-term effects of bariatric surgery on liver injury in patients without advanced disease. Gastroenterology 2009;137:532–40.
71. Mosko JD, Nguyen GC. Increased perioperative mortality following bariatric surgery among patients with cirrhosis. Clin Gastroenterol Hepatol 2011;9:897–901.

Helping Patients with Gastroparesis

Frances U. Onyimba, MD[a], John O. Clarke, MD[b],*

KEYWORDS

- Gastroparesis • Nausea • Vomiting • Prokinetics • Gastric electrical stimulation

KEY POINTS

- Diagnosis of gastroparesis hinges on identification of abnormal gastric emptying in the absence of obstructive etiologies.
- Treatment of gastroparesis can be tailored to the patient's individual symptoms and desires using lifestyle modification, medications, complementary therapy, and endoscopic/surgical options in select cases.
- Medical therapy consists of antiemetics, prokinetics, neuromodulators, and accommodation-enhancers.
- Endoscopic and surgical therapy can be directed to pyloric disruption, gastric electrical stimulation, resection, and venting/bypass.

INTRODUCTION

Gastroparesis is a chronic and, in severe cases, life-impairing condition that has been increasingly recognized in our patient populations. The heterogeneous pathophysiology, etiologies, and symptomatology of gastroparesis may present a diagnostic and therapeutic challenge to practitioners. In this review, the authors offer clinical pearls to help clinicians identify and manage patients, and cover the broad medical options as well as emerging endoscopic options for the management of the disorder and highlight the prospects of an exciting future with mechanism-based therapy.

WHAT IS GASTROPARESIS?

Gastroparesis is a chronic condition characterized by the presence of upper gastrointestinal (GI) symptoms and delayed gastric emptying in the absence of mechanical obstruction.[1]

Disclosure Statement: The authors have no relevant conflicts of interest.
a Department of Medicine, Division of Gastroenterology, University of California San Diego, 9500 Gillman Drive, #0956, La Jolla, CA 92093, USA; b Department of Medicine, Division of Gastroenterology and Hepatology, Stanford University, 300 Pasteur Drive, MC 5244, Stanford, CA 94305, USA
* Corresponding author.
E-mail address: john.clarke@stanford.edu

Med Clin N Am 103 (2019) 71–87
https://doi.org/10.1016/j.mcna.2018.08.013
0025-7125/19/© 2018 Elsevier Inc. All rights reserved.

medical.theclinics.com

Pathophysiology

After a meal is ingested, the stomach must execute 3 basic functions: accommodation, trituration, and coordinated emptying. Propulsive forces from contractions of the gastric antrum and tone of the gastric fundus overcome resistance from the pylorus to empty solid food into the small bowel. These functions are regulated by an interplay among the gastric smooth muscle, Interstitial Cells of Cajal (ICC), enteric nervous system, and extrinsic innervation. Decreased fundic tone, antroduodenal dyscoordination, weak antral contractions, and abnormal duodenal feedback all may contribute to abnormal gastric emptying and symptom generation.[2]

Etiology

Although diabetes mellitus is recognized as the classic risk factor for gastroparesis, it is important to note that the most common presentation in the United States is idiopathic (35.6%). Most patients with idiopathic gastroparesis are young or middle-aged women and have neuronal and ICC degeneration. Some have hypothesized that idiopathic gastroparesis may occur as a postviral syndrome, because up to 23% of patients with idiopathic gastroparesis were observed to have a viral prodrome.[3,4] Other common etiologies of gastroparesis include diabetes (28.8%), postsurgical (13%), neurologic disease (7.5%), connective tissue disease (4.8%), postinfectious (8.2%), and miscellaneous (6.2%).[5] Data suggest that up to 50% of patients with type 1 diabetes and 30% of patients with type 2 diabetes have gastroparesis.[6] Acute departures from normoglycemia change antral contractility, pyloric pressure waves, and gastric myoelectrical activity leading to reversibly delayed gastric emptying.[7,8] With longstanding hyperglycemia, damage to the enteric nervous system dampens antral phasic contractility leading to delayed transit. Postsurgical gastroparesis develops in response to vagal nerve injury during foregut surgery. Concurrent distal gastric resection may further worsen gastric stasis due to loss of trituration and propulsive antral forces.[9,10] Other relevant causes include medication-induced gastroparesis, gastric dysmotility due to neurodegenerative diseases, autoimmune disease such as systemic sclerosis, and undiagnosed paraneoplastic processes.

Prevalence and Epidemiology

Although firm prevalence data are lacking, studies based on symptoms of gastroparesis suggest a prevalence of approximately 1.5% to 3.0% in the general population, with increase over the past 20 years.[11,12] Women account for up to 70% of the affected population. Younger patients are also disproportionately affected. Interestingly, elderly patients (>65 years old) constitute a large percentage of diagnoses, accounting for approximately 20% of patients with gastroparesis.[13]

Although most management occurs in the outpatient setting, the number of hospitalizations for gastroparesis has catapulted over the past decade. A study by Nusrat and Bielfeldt[13] found that annual hospitalizations for gastroparesis increased more than 18-fold, from 918 to 16,736 between 1994 and 2009. Admissions for gastroparesis have the longest length of stay and highest associated charges of the 5 most common upper GI conditions leading to hospitalization.[14] Limited data are available regarding the prognosis and natural history of gastroparesis; however, available data from tertiary referral centers show mortality of 4% to 12%.[5,15] Increased mortality, when found, is typically due to cardiovascular complications in diabetic patients.[11]

Symptoms and Clinical Presentation

Patients with gastroparesis classically present with nausea (92%), vomiting (84%), early satiety (60%), and fullness/bloating (75%).[5] Earlier studies underestimated the pain component of gastroparesis, to a point that it is not included on the Gastroparesis Cardinal Symptom Index. However, there has been increasing recognition that abdominal pain is a dominant symptom in many patients with gastroparesis and in fact is reported in 90% of affected patients.[16,17] Symptoms are variable and may be mild or occur in debilitating flares.

Differential Diagnosis

As symptoms may be nonspecific, the differential diagnosis of gastroparesis is broad and includes gastric outlet obstruction, peptic ulcer disease, and gastrointestinal cancer, as well as a myriad of functional GI disorders including functional dyspepsia, cyclical vomiting syndrome, chronic nausea and vomiting syndrome, cannabinoid hyperemesis syndrome, and eating disorders. Although clues can be elicited from a careful history, diagnostic tests are almost always required to exclude other entities and confirm diagnosis.

HOW TO DIAGNOSE GASTROPARESIS

A thorough history and physical examination help to identify the presence of characteristic symptoms of gastroparesis and exclude alternative diagnoses. Once the syndrome is suspected, an upper endoscopy is necessary to rule out mechanical obstruction. Although an upper GI series may suggest the diagnosis, there is a limited role for imaging in the workup for gastroparesis and delayed emptying should be confirmed by gastric transit testing. Diagnostic options for gastroparesis are summarized in **Table 1**.

Gastric Scintigraphy

A 4-hour solid-phase gastric emptying scintigraphy test is considered the gold standard for diagnosis.[1,18] The test is a nuclear medicine study that detects transit of a technetium-99–labeled meal typically consisting of an egg, toast, and water. Images are captured at 0, 1, 2, and 4 hours and results reported as percentage of food retained at each time point. Greater than 60% retention at 2 hours and greater than 90% retention at 4 hours are considered abnormal results.[19] Other solid-phase protocols, including 60-minute, 90-minute, and 120-minute protocols have been shown to be less reliable and are not clinically recommended. Although solid-phase gastric emptying scintigraphy is considered the gold standard, there are data that suggest liquid scintigraphy may also have a role in select patients[20] and the National Institutes of Health (NIH) Gastroparesis Clinical Research Consortium (GCRC) is currently investigating the diagnostic characteristics of a combined solid/liquid scintigraphic study.

Wireless Motility Capsule Study

The wireless motility capsule was approved by the Food and Drug Administration (FDA) for the evaluation of delayed gastric transit in 2006 and offers a nonradioactive ambulatory alternative to gastric scintigraphy. A 2.6-cm orally digested capsule collects and transmits luminal pH, temperature, and pressure data to a recorder worn by the patient. The gastric emptying time is then calculated using a combination of pH and temperature profiles. When compared with gastric scintigraphy in healthy patients and patients with gastroparesis, a cutoff of 5 hours for normal gastric emptying correlates well with gastric scintigraphy (correlation coefficient of 0.73 with 4-hour

Table 1
Comparison of diagnostic studies to evaluate gastroparesis

	Method	Parameter Measured	Validated	Advantages	Disadvantages
Gastric emptying studies					
Gastric scintigraphy	4-h study of radiolabeled solid meal	Gastric transit time	Yes	"Gold standard"	Radiation exposure
Breath testing	$^{13}CO_2$ measurement after ingested meal	Gastric transit time	Yes	Noninvasive	Relies on normal intestinal absorption and liver metabolism
Wireless motility capsule	Oral ingested capsule that measures pH, temperature, and pressure	Gastric transit time	Yes	Noninvasive, explores whole gut motility	Contraindicated in patients with strictures, single time point
Other					
Electrogastrography	External electrodes	Myoelectrical activity	No	Noninvasive	Limited utility in management
Antroduodenal manometry	Intraluminal catheter with pressure transducers	Antral contractions, pyloric pressure	No	Distinguishes myopathic vs neuropathic processes	Invasive, requires expert interpretation
EndoFLIP	Transpyloric balloon catheter with pressure sensors	Pyloric distensibility	No	May identify patients for pyloric intervention	Invasive, normative data unclear

gastric scintigraphy).[21] Capsule studies are contraindicated in patients with known gastrointestinal strictures and relatively contraindicated in patients with implantable electronic devices, although no data have shown significant risk with the latter.

Breath Testing

Gastric emptying breath testing (GEBT) is a nonradioactive, noninvasive means to assess gastric emptying that was FDA approved in 2015. It uses a meal mixed with stable isotope carbon-13–labeled Spirulina. As the Spirulina passes to the duodenum, it is absorbed and metabolized to $^{13}CO_2$, which is measured in end-tidal breaths by mass spectrometry. The $^{13}CO_2/^{12}CO_2$ ratio is then used to determine the gastric emptying rate. GEBT is used in ambulatory settings and has been validated against gastric scintigraphy with greater than 89% specificity.[22] The test is not recommended in patients with pancreas or liver disease due to altered metabolism.

Before any transit test, patients are instructed to discontinue medications such as opiates and anticholinergics, as well as prokinetic agents, which can cause false-positive results and false-negative results, respectively. The role of transit testing during hyperglycemia in diabetic patients has been debated, but generally should be avoided, as hyperglycemia can cause delayed transit.[23]

Complementary Nontransit Testing

Electrogastrography (EGG) provides a noninvasive assessment of gastric myoelectrical activity. Electrodes placed over the epigastrium record electrical activity of the gastric pacemaker cells in the muscular layer of the gastric body and antrum. Dysrhythmias, notably bradygastria and tachygastria, have been described in patients with nausea, vomiting, and gastroparesis.[24] Although there are limited data that correction of these dysrhythmias may improve symptoms independent of gastric emptying, at present EGG remains primarily a research tool.[25]

Antroduodenal manometry involves transpyloric placement of a catheter with pressure transducers to measure antral and small bowel contractility. In patients with gastroparesis, this provides reliable characterization of pyloric activity, often detecting decreased antral contractions or increased pyloric pressure. Although perhaps useful in the delineation of neuropathic versus myopathic causes of gastric and small bowel stasis, the procedure is not routinely used in the clinical evaluation of gastroparesis at most medical centers.[26]

The most recent advancement in diagnostic testing is the functional lumen imaging probe (FLIP). During this procedure, a fluid-filled highly compliant balloon is positioned across the pylorus and gradually inflated. Through use of impedance planimetry, pyloric diameter and distensibility can be directly measured. Limited data suggest that subsets of gastroparesis may have altered pyloric dynamics[27,28] and that pyloric-directed therapy may be more beneficial in patients with decreased pyloric compliance.[29] Although further data are needed to establish the role of FLIP in the evaluation of gastroparesis, this device is actively being evaluated as a predictor of response to pyloric-directed therapy.

KEY CONTROVERSIES
Distinction Between Gastroparesis and Functional Dyspepsia

Many of the symptoms of gastroparesis, particularly nausea, vomiting, and epigastric pain, demonstrate significant overlap with functional dyspepsia (FD), making the symptoms relatively nonspecific for diagnosis. Gastroparesis and FD also share impaired physiologic processes, including visceral hypersensitivity, impaired accommodation, and gastric dysrhythmia.[30] Hasler and colleagues[31] in the GCRC showed that most patients with gastroparesis meet diagnostic criteria for FD. Conversely, approximately 30% of patients with FD have been shown to have delayed gastric emptying.[32] These overlaps have generated debate over whether there is a meaningful distinction between the 2 disorders.

Lack of Correlation Between Symptoms and Gastric Emptying

Interestingly, trials using prokinetics have found no clear correlation between changes in gastric emptying and symptom improvement. A meta-analysis conducted by Janssen and colleagues[33] evaluated 34 trials comparing symptom improvement (SI) and gastric emptying using various prokinetics. Although studies demonstrated a concomitant improvement in symptoms and gastric emptying and a trend toward SI and gastric emptying acceleration, no individual study showed significant correlation between SI and gastric emptying.[33] This questions the link between symptom relief and improved gastric emptying. This ongoing debate and discrepancy between SI and gastric emptying may be explained by the notion of overlap between gastroparesis and FD and the role of other mechanisms, such as impaired gastric accommodation and visceral hypersensitivity. However, it is certainly possible that gastric emptying is not the cause of symptoms in patients with gastroparesis but rather an indirect marker of gastric dysfunction.

HOW TO TREAT YOUR PATIENTS WITH GASTROPARESIS

As detailed previously, there is not a strong correlation between symptom severity and gastric emptying. Therefore, treatment should not be tailored to improved gastric emptying alone and symptom relief is the primary goal of management.

Lifestyle Modification

Lifestyle modifications, especially dietary changes, are invaluable in the fight for symptom relief. Smaller, lower calorie meals are associated with shorter emptying times, whereas high-fat and high-fiber meals are associated with prolonged emptying times and increased symptomatology.[34,35] Based on these physiologic principles, guidelines recommend small meals with low fat and fiber content. Frequent meals (up to 4–5 times per day) allow for adequate caloric intake while decreasing sensation of fullness. Liquid emptying is often preserved in patients with delayed solid-phase emptying, making meals of liquid or pureed consistency easier to tolerate, particularly during flares. Alcohol use and tobacco smoking decrease antral contractility and worsen gastric emptying and should be avoided.[36]

In addition to dietary changes, patients presenting with complaints of gastroparesis should undergo medication reconciliation. Medication such as opiates, anticholinergics, diphenhydramine, tricyclic antidepressants, GLP-1 analogs, and calcium channel blockers can delay gastric emptying and should be minimized. Similarly, glycemic control should be optimized in patients with diabetes. A recent study from the GCRC demonstrated improved quality of life and decreased symptoms in patients with diabetic gastroparesis started on a subcutaneous insulin pump with improved glycemic control.[37]

MEDICAL THERAPY

Medical therapy is usually the next step for patients who remain symptomatic despite lifestyle and dietary modification. Options for medical therapy fall into several broad categories: antiemetics, prokinetics, accommodation-enhancers, and neuromodulators. An overview of the medications used for gastroparesis is summarized in **Table 2**.

Antiemetics

There are limited data with regard to the use of specific antiemetics for patients with gastroparesis. However, in practice, antiemetics are used commonly based on data extrapolated from oncology literature. Ondansetron (a 5-HT$_3$ antagonist) and promethazine (a phenothiazine derivative and H$_1$ antagonist) are the most commonly prescribed agents. Although antiemetics have no significant effect on gastric emptying, they do help control nausea, which is often the dominant symptom. Sedation and extrapyramidal effects may occur, with individual adverse effects varying based on the agent used. Antihistamines, specifically H$_1$ receptor blockers, such as meclizine, have limited literature supporting use in gastroparesis, but are empirically used as antiemetics due to their effects in motion sickness and postsurgical nausea. Transdermal scopolamine, a muscarinic cholinergic receptor antagonist, is approved for motion sickness but often used off label for nausea in gastroparesis. Transdermal granisetron is a 5-HT$_3$ receptor antagonist initially developed for chemotherapy-induced nausea and vomiting, which has recently been shown to be effective in relieving nausea and vomiting in patients with gastroparesis specifically.[38] Aprepitant, a neurokinin-1 receptor antagonist, is approved for use in chemotherapy-induced nausea. A recently published placebo-controlled randomized controlled trial by the GCRC failed to meet the primary outcome, but found decreased severity of nausea and vomiting in patients with gastroparesis or gastroparesislike syndrome.[39]

For many of these agents, cost and formulary restrictions limit availability. In our practice, we often will start with oral ondansetron or promethazine, based on patient preference and prior experience. If patients have frequent vomiting, rectally administered promethazine can be an option that guarantees drug delivery. Transdermal granisetron is also an attractive option if covered by insurance, because the patch avoids oral routes of absorption and can be applied for a week.

Prokinetics

The use of prokinetics for the treatment of gastroparesis was established after early studies with metoclopramide demonstrated superiority to placebo for improved gastric emptying, nausea, vomiting, and fullness in patients with diabetic, idiopathic, and postsurgical gastroparesis.[40,41] Metoclopramide is a prokinetic and antiemetic agent that acts on central and peripheral D$_2$ receptors, as well as 5-HT$_4$ receptors, to improve antral contractions, gastric dysrhythmias, and antroduodenal coordination. It remains the only FDA-approved treatment of gastroparesis, but carries an FDA-issued black box warning due to the risk of tardive dyskinesia. The risk of tardive dyskinesia is now believed to be less than 1%; nevertheless, guidelines recommend limiting metoclopramide use to a maximum of 3 months at the lowest possible dose.[42] In our practice, we will often use liquid metoclopramide and will start at 5 mg per dose, increasing if necessary and no adverse effects.

Domperidone is a peripheral D$_2$ receptor antagonist with prokinetic and antiemetic properties. Studies suggest similar efficacy to metoclopramide, but with a lower side-effect profile, allowing for dose titration.[43,44] Adverse effects include hyperprolactinemia and potential QT prolongation. Domperidone is not FDA approved and is unlikely to be approved in the future due to concerns regarding cardiac toxicity. However, it can be obtained through an Investigational New Drug Application from the FDA, although the paperwork and data monitoring involved are onerous.

Table 2
Summary of medical options for gastroparesis

	Mechanism	Recommended	Evidence in Gastroparesis	Limitations
Antiemetics				
Phenothiazines (chlorpromazine, promethazine)	Multiple: $D_2/H_1/M_1$	Yes	None	QT prolongation, somnolence
Scopolamine	Muscarinic (M_1)	Yes	None	Drying effects, anticholinergic
Antihistamines	Histamine (H_1)	Yes	None	Drowsiness
Serotonin antagonists (ondansetron, granisetron)	5-HT_3	Yes	Yes (granisetron)	Headache, constipation, QT prolongation
Aprepitant	Neurokinin-1	Case-by-case	Limited	Cost, fatigue, headache, neutropenia
Prokinetics				
Metoclopramide	Dopamine (D_2), Serotonin (5-HT_4)	Yes	Yes	Extrapyramidal effects, anxiety, restlessness, tardive dyskinesia

Domperidone	Dopamine (D_2)	Not approved by the Food and Drug Administration (FDA) but available via IND	Yes	QT prolongation, hyperprolactinemia
Erythromycin	Motilin	Best for acute use	Limited	Tachyphylaxis, ototoxicity, QT prolongation
Cisapride	Serotonin (5-HT_4)	Not FDA approved	Yes	Sudden cardiac death
Prucalopride	Serotonin (5-HT_4)	Not FDA approved	No	Minimal: thought to have no arrhythmogenic effects
Neuromodulators				
Tricyclic antidepressants	Serotonin/Norepinephrine	Case-by-case (abdominal pain)	Limited	Somnolence, constipation, dry mouth
Mirtazapine	Tetracyclic antidepressant	Case-by-case (nausea)	Limited	Drowsiness, weight gain
Other				
Buspirone	Serotonin (5-HT_1)	Case-by-case (postprandial bloating)	Limited (data for functional dyspepsia)	Dizziness, drowsiness, headache

Other prokinetic drugs include serotonergic drugs, motilin receptor agonists and ghrelin receptor agonists. Erythromycin and azithromycin are macrolide antibiotics that stimulate the motilin receptor to promote gastroduodenal motility. Erythromycin has been shown to be a potent prokinetic, but data on clinical improvement are limited. The development of tachyphylaxis and QT prolongation limit the ambulatory use of erythromycin. In our practice, this has not been an effective option for most symptomatic patients. Prucalopride is a 5-HT$_4$ receptor agonist approved in Europe and Canada for treatment of chronic idiopathic constipation. It is not yet FDA approved, but is scheduled to be presented to the FDA within a year of this writing. Data show improved gastric emptying in healthy subjects and suggest a role in gastroparesis, but more studies are needed.[45] Cisapride is an older 5-HT$_4$ receptor antagonist with gastroprokinetic properties, initially approved for heartburn. However, the medication was removed from the US market in 2000, due to effects of QT prolongation and concern for cardiac dysrhythmias. This is available for compassionate use but does seem to have more significant cardiac risk than other available options. There are minimal data on the use of selective serotonin reuptake inhibitors in the management of gastroparesis, but data support improvement in gastric emptying and increased accommodation in FD and we occasionally will use them in our practice. The response to treatment for any prokinetic agent should be evaluated clinically rather than by repeat gastric emptying studies.

Buspirone

Data suggest that approximately 30% of patients with gastroparesis have impaired accommodation.[30] Buspirone is a 5-HT$_1$ receptor agonist that increases gastric accommodation in healthy controls.[46] Although not explicitly studied in gastroparesis, in a double-blinded, placebo-controlled, crossover trial, buspirone improved symptoms and gastric accommodation in patients with FD, while delaying liquid gastric emptying.[47] Its use has been suggested in patients with gastroparesis and in our practice we often use it to treat patients with gastroparesis and prominent postprandial bloating.

Neuromodulators

Low-dose tricyclic antidepressants (TCAs) have demonstrated efficacy in improving nausea, vomiting, and abdominal pain in patients with FD, as well as idiopathic and diabetic gastroparesis. In a retrospective analysis by investigators at Washington University, TCAs improved chronic vomiting in patients with diabetes who failed to respond to prokinetics.[48] Given these data in tandem with clinical experience, the GCRC evaluated nortriptyline versus placebo in a large randomized controlled trial in patients with idiopathic gastroparesis. Unfortunately, the study did not meet its primary endpoint and use of nortriptyline did not improve overall symptoms when compared with placebo.[49] Although this study dampened enthusiasm for TCA use, we still use TCAs in our practice on a case-by-case basis primarily when pain is a dominant symptom. Nortriptyline and desipramine have a less potent anticholinergic effect than older TCAs and may be better tolerated.

Mirtazapine is an atypical antidepressant noted to have a prominent central antiemetic effect that has been used clinically for treatment of gastroparesis symptoms. In a recent open-label prospective pilot study from Temple University, mirtazapine significantly improved nausea and vomiting in gastroparetic patients at weeks 2 and 4; however, side effects were noted in 20% of patients.[50] In a recent randomized controlled trial evaluating mirtazapine in FD, mirtazapine significantly improved early satiation, quality of life, nutrient tolerance, and weight loss.[32] In our practice, we will often use this at low dose nightly in patients with nausea-dominant symptoms. We generally will start at 7.5 mg for the first week and then increase to 15.0 mg nightly thereafter if symptoms continue and side effects are minimal.

ALTERNATIVE AND COMPLEMENTARY THERAPIES

Acupuncture is the most studied alternative therapy for gastroparesis. Stimulation of various pressure points in the wrist and below the patella have been shown to alleviate nausea and increase gastric motility via vagal stimulation and serotonin modulation.[51] A randomized controlled trial in 19 patients with diabetic gastroparesis found that electroacupuncture improved symptoms and gastric emptying up to 2 weeks after treatment.[52] In our practice, we often recommend it given limited approved treatment options, high patient acceptance, and excellent safety profile. Ginger is another alternative option for patients who wish to avoid medical therapy. It has never been studied formally in gastroparesis, but has shown to reduce nausea from other conditions and accelerate gastric emptying. Iberogast is an over-the-counter liquid herbal preparation used in clinical practice for FD and gastroparesis. A placebo-controlled, crossover study in 103 patients with FD and gastroparesis demonstrated improvement in symptoms without effect on gastric emptying.[53] No literature currently supports the use of marijuana or magnetic bracelets in the treatment of gastroparesis, although anecdotal reports suggest benefit in some patients. Patients may also benefit from psychotherapy and hypnosis.

ENDOSCOPIC AND SURGICAL THERAPY

Given the limited medical options available to treat gastroparesis and that there is only 1 FDA-approved medication at present (metoclopramide), there has been significant interest in endoscopic and surgical options. Generally, these options fall into 4 categories: pyloric disruption, electrical stimulation, venting/bypass, and resection.

Pyloric Therapies

Botulinum toxin is a potent neuromuscular inhibitor used in the treatment of spastic muscle disorders. The first description of intrapyloric botulinum toxin for the treatment of refractory gastroparesis was described in 1998. Several small open-label studies demonstrated 30% to 60% improvement in symptoms and solid-phase gastric emptying after pyloric botulinum toxin injections.[54,55] Unfortunately, both randomized controlled trials performed to date have shown no significant improvement in symptoms or gastric emptying compared with sham injections; however, both were small studies and concerns have been raised about their power.[56,57] In the absence of randomized controlled trial data showing efficacy with botulinum toxin, it is hard to endorse this therapy for routine use; however, there do appear to be subgroups who may benefit from this therapy and it is an option on a case-by-case basis.[58] In our practice, we will often attempt botulinum toxin once in patients with refractory symptoms who have failed other options. Clinical response to botulinum toxin may also serve a prognostic role when more aggressive pyloric therapies are under discussion.

Transpyloric stent placement is another option for patients with gastroparesis with pyloric dysfunction. A 3-patient case series from 2013 and a retrospective analysis of 30 patients in 2015 showed subjective improvement in symptoms of gastroparesis and gastric emptying in up to 75% of patients.[59,60] Stent migration is a concern, and at present this therapy remains largely investigational; however, much like botulinum toxin injection, it may have a role as a bridging therapy or prognostic role in patients being considered for more permanent pyloric disruption.

Per oral endoscopic pyloric myotomy (also referred to as G-POEM or POP) is a new advanced endoscopic procedure for mechanical disruption of the pylorus. The first successful human application of submucosal tunneling for refractory gastroparesis was described by Khashab and colleagues in 2013.[61] Since then, several small series have been published with promising results. A recently retrospective review of 30 patients and a multicenter international cohort of 33 patients with refractory gastroparesis undergoing G-POEM showed 70% to 85% improvement in symptoms and improvement in quality of life at 1 year with a low rate of adverse events.[62–64] However, no randomized trials have been performed using G-POEM to date and further multicenter data are needed to determine where this therapy fits in the gastroparesis treatment algorithm and clarify which patients may most likely benefit.

Pyloroplasty is a surgical drainage procedure that increases the pyloric diameter for patients with refractory gastroparesis.[65] A retrospective study of pyloroplasty in 46 patients with gastroparesis showed SI in 90% of patients based on a validated symptom scale and 60% with normalization of gastric emptying.[66] Similarly, a retrospective analysis of 117 patients with presumed gastroparesis by Shada and colleagues[67] showed improved mean symptom severity in 8 of 9 domains. Overall, pyloroplasty is less invasive and less morbid than larger resections, such as a partial or complete gastrectomy; however, similar to G-POEM, randomized data are needed to determine relative efficacy compared with other therapies and guide patient selection. No trials to date have compared G-POEM with pyloroplasty.

Gastric Stimulator

The gastric electrical stimulator (GES) is available via a Humanitarian Device Exemption from the FDA for refractory gastroparesis. The stimulator is surgically implanted into the anterior abdominal wall with electrodes placed on the gastric antrum to deliver high-frequency electrical stimulation. The device was evaluated in 2 key landmark randomized controlled trials. Abell and colleagues[68] in 2003 evaluated the device in a crossover study in which patients were randomized to 1 month on/off stimulation and then kept on stimulation for the conclusion of a 12-month period. Although the patients significantly improved over the course of the year, the on/off periods could not be separated. In a second landmark randomized controlled trial, McCallum and colleagues[69] evaluated patients with GES placement over 1 year. Again, the patients significantly improved over the year; however, the on/off stimulation periods could not be separated. In our practice, we do offer GES to select patients with nausea-predominant symptoms who are refractory to other therapies; however, clinical response is highly variable and more data are needed to guide patient selection.

More recently, a temporary endoscopically placed gastric stimulator was developed for transmucosal stimulation by Abell and colleagues.[70] Two studies, including a double-blinded randomized crossover trial, did not meet the criteria for success, defined as greater than 50% improvement in symptoms, using the temporary gastric stimulation. However, short-term improvement with temporary gastric stimulator placement correlated with long-term benefits from a traditional gastric electrical stimulation.[71] The role of temporary endoscopic stimulation remains uncertain; however, if it can predict clinical response to permanent stimulator implantation, then it may allow more tailored selection of GES placement and has the potential to significantly impact patient management.

Gastrostomy Tube Placement

A small minority of patients with refractory gastroparesis are unable to tolerate oral intake and develop weight loss, recurrent dehydration, and electrolyte imbalance requiring supplemental nutrition. In such patients, postpyloric enteral feeding with a jejunostomy tube is recommended over parenteral nutrition.[23] Jejunostomy tube placement may reduce hospital admissions and maximize nutritional status, but has no effect on quality of life or symptom relief.[72] Venting gastrostomy tube placement for intermittent decompression has also been reported; however, in our practice this generally does not relieve symptoms other than in rare cases and is not routinely recommended.

Gastrectomy

Subtotal gastrectomy has been recommended by some authorities for refractory gastroparesis. Although it may have a role in select patients with postvagotomy gastroparesis, we do not recommend it for patients in other subgroups. Although gastroparesis is often defined based on gastric emptying, the mechanisms at play in most patients lead to systemic dysfunction, and our personal experience with subtotal gastrectomy for these patients has not been encouraging.

SUPPORT GROUPS AND IMPORTANCE OF SOCIAL SUPPORT

Because of the distressing nature of the disease, patients may benefit from a multidisciplinary approach and social support. G-PACT, the Gastroparesis Patient Association for Cures and Treatment, is a volunteer-based organization dedicated to the care of patients suffering from intestinal motility disorders, including gastroparesis, chronic intestinal pseudo obstruction, and colonic inertia. The organization provides educational resources, support programs, and patient advocacy programs. The NIH GCRC was established to advance research on the natural history, diagnosis, and treatment of gastroparesis. Patients are able to enroll in clinical trials through the consortium, gain access to studies, and find a support group. Other support groups exist in local chapters or via social media. It is our opinion that an important aspect of patient care is ensuring that they are appropriately connected to other affected patients.

FUTURE DIRECTIONS

The field of gastroparesis is rapidly en flux and there are significant changes on the horizon. There is increasing recognition that gastroparesis is likely a heterogeneous syndrome composed of numerous distinct subgroups, with different pathophysiology and treatment response. This recognition has been spurred by the work of the NIH GCRC and the increased access to deep tissue pathology through advanced endoscopic techniques. Better understanding of underlying mechanisms holds the promise of tailored therapy directed at the underlying process. Novel drugs are in the pipeline, with relamorelin now in phase III trials and showing particular promise. Nonmedical therapies, in particular pyloric-directed therapies, will likely be defined further in upcoming years, allowing better patient selection. We suspect that the way gastroparesis is approached 15 years from now will be quite different from how we approach it today.

SUMMARY

Gastroparesis is a disease in evolution. Diagnosis hinges on identification of impaired gastric emptying, with other nontransit studies such as FLIP providing supportive information. Treatment at present consists of diet/lifestyle, medical, alternative, endoscopic, and surgical options. Choice of which agent to use is based on individual patient preferences and local treatment patterns and expertise.

REFERENCES

1. Pasricha PJ, Parkman HP. Gastroparesis: definitions and diagnosis. Gastroenterol Clin North Am 2015;44:1–7.
2. Parkman HP, Hasler WL, Fisher RS, et al. American Gastroenterological Association technical review on the diagnosis and treatment of gastroparesis. Gastroenterology 2004;127:1592–622.
3. Oh JJ, Kim CH. Gastroparesis after a presumed viral illness: clinical and laboratory features and natural history. Mayo Clin Proc 1990;65:636–42.
4. Bityutskiy LP, Soykan I, McCallum RW. Viral gastroparesis: a subgroup of idiopathic gastroparesis—clinical characteristics and long-term outcomes. Am J Gastroenterol 1997;92:1501–4.
5. Soykan I, Sivri B, Sarosiek I, et al. Demography, clinical characteristics, psychological and abuse profiles, treatment, and long-term follow-up of patients with gastroparesis. Dig Dis Sci 1998;43:2398–404.
6. Maleki D, Locke GR, Camilleri M, et al. Gastrointestinal tract symptoms among persons with diabetes mellitus in the community. Arch Intern Med 2000;160: 2808–16.
7. Fraser RJ, Horowitz M, Maddox AF, et al. Hyperglycaemia slows gastric emptying in type 1 (insulin-dependent) diabetes mellitus. Diabetologia 1990;33:675–80.
8. Bharucha AE, Kudva Y, Basu A, et al. Relationship between glycemic control and gastric emptying in poorly controlled type 2 diabetes. Clin Gastroenterol Hepatol 2015;13:466–76.e1.
9. Eagon JC, Miedema BW, Kelly KA. Postgastrectomy syndromes. Surg Clin North Am 1992;72:445–65.
10. Horowitz M, Cook DJ, Collins PJ, et al. Measurement of gastric emptying after gastric bypass surgery using radionuclides. Br J Surg 1982;69:655–7.
11. Jung HK, Choung RS, Locke GR, et al. The incidence, prevalence, and outcomes of patients with gastroparesis in Olmsted County, Minnesota, from 1996 to 2006. Gastroenterology 2009;136:1225–33.
12. Rey E, Choung RS, Schleck CD, et al. Prevalence of hidden gastroparesis in the community: the gastroparesis "iceberg". J Neurogastroenterol Motil 2012;18: 34–42.
13. Nusrat S, Bielefeldt K. Gastroparesis on the rise: incidence vs awareness? Neurogastroenterol Motil 2013;25:16–22.
14. Wang YR, Fisher RS, Parkman HP. Gastroparesis-related hospitalizations in the United States: trends, characteristics, and outcomes, 1995-2004. Am J Gastroenterol 2008;103:313–22.
15. Dudekula A, O'Connell M, Bielefeldt K. Hospitalizations and testing in gastroparesis. J Gastroenterol Hepatol 2011;26:1275–82.
16. Hoogerwerf WA, Pasricha PJ, Kalloo AN, et al. Pain: the overlooked symptom in gastroparesis. Am J Gastroenterol 1999;94:1029–33.
17. Cherian D, Sachdeva P, Fisher RS, et al. Abdominal pain is a frequent symptom of gastroparesis. Clin Gastroenterol Hepatol 2010;8:676–81.
18. Abell TL, Camilleri M, Donohoe K, et al. Consensus recommendations for gastric emptying scintigraphy: a joint report of the American Neurogastroenterology and

Motility Society and the Society of Nuclear Medicine. Am J Gastroenterol 2008; 103:753–63.

19. Tougas G, Eaker EY, Abell TL, et al. Assessment of gastric emptying using a low fat meal: establishment of international control values. Am J Gastroenterol 2000; 95:1456–62.

20. Ziessman HA, Chander A, Clarke JO, et al. The added diagnostic value of liquid gastric emptying compared with solid emptying alone. J Nucl Med 2009;50: 726–31.

21. Kuo B, McCallum RW, Koch KL, et al. Comparison of gastric emptying of a non-digestible capsule to a radio-labelled meal in healthy and gastroparetic subjects. Aliment Pharmacol Ther 2008;27:186–96.

22. Bharucha AE, Camilleri M, Veil E, et al. Comprehensive assessment of gastric emptying with a stable isotope breath test. Neurogastroenterol Motil 2013;25: e60–9.

23. Camilleri M, Parkman HP, Shafi MA, et al. Clinical guideline: management of gastroparesis. Am J Gastroenterol 2013;108:18–37 [quiz: 38].

24. Chen JD, Lin Z, Pan J, et al. Abnormal gastric myoelectrical activity and delayed gastric emptying in patients with symptoms suggestive of gastroparesis. Dig Dis Sci 1996;41:1538–45.

25. Koch KL. Electrogastrography: physiological basis and clinical application in diabetic gastropathy. Diabetes Technol Ther 2001;3:51–62.

26. Patcharatrakul T, Gonlachanvit S. Technique of functional and motility test: how to perform antroduodenal manometry. J Neurogastroenterol Motil 2013;19:395–404.

27. Malik Z, Sankineni A, Parkman HP. Assessing pyloric sphincter pathophysiology using EndoFLIP in patients with gastroparesis. Neurogastroenterol Motil 2015;27: 524–31.

28. Snape WJ, Lin MS, Agarwal N, et al. Evaluation of the pylorus with concurrent intraluminal pressure and EndoFLIP in patients with nausea and vomiting. Neurogastroenterol Motil 2016;28:758–64.

29. Gourcerol G, Tissier F, Melchior C, et al. Impaired fasting pyloric compliance in gastroparesis and the therapeutic response to pyloric dilatation. Aliment Pharmacol Ther 2015;41:360–7.

30. Karamanolis G, Caenepeel P, Arts J, et al. Association of the predominant symptom with clinical characteristics and pathophysiological mechanisms in functional dyspepsia. Gastroenterology 2006;130:296–303.

31. Hasler WL, Parkman HP, Wilson LA, et al. Psychological dysfunction is associated with symptom severity but not disease etiology or degree of gastric retention in patients with gastroparesis. Am J Gastroenterol 2010;105:2357–67.

32. Tack J, Carbone F. Functional dyspepsia and gastroparesis. Curr Opin Gastroenterol 2017;33:446–54.

33. Janssen P, Harris MS, Jones M, et al. The relation between symptom improvement and gastric emptying in the treatment of diabetic and idiopathic gastroparesis. Am J Gastroenterol 2013;108:1382–91.

34. Moore JG, Christian PE, Brown JA, et al. Influence of meal weight and caloric content on gastric emptying of meals in man. Dig Dis Sci 1984;29:513–9.

35. Homko CJ, Duffy F, Friedenberg FK, et al. Effect of dietary fat and food consistency on gastroparesis symptoms in patients with gastroparesis. Neurogastroenterol Motil 2015;27:501–8.

36. Bujanda L. The effects of alcohol consumption upon the gastrointestinal tract. Am J Gastroenterol 2000;95:3374–82.

37. Calles-Escandón J, Koch KL, Hasler WL, et al. Glucose sensor-augmented continuous subcutaneous insulin infusion in patients with diabetic gastroparesis: an open-label pilot prospective study. PLoS One 2018;13:e0194759.

38. Midani D, Parkman HP. Granisetron transdermal system for treatment of symptoms of gastroparesis: a prescription registry study. J Neurogastroenterol Motil 2016;22:650–5.

39. Pasricha PJ, Yates KP, Sarosiek I, et al. Aprepitant has mixed effects on nausea and reduces other symptoms in patients with gastroparesis and related disorders. Gastroenterology 2018;154:65–76.e1.

40. Brownlee M, Kroopf SS. Letter: metoclopramide for gastroparesis diabeticorum. N Engl J Med 1974;291:1257–8.

41. Longstreth GF, Malagelada JR, Kelly KA. Metoclopramide stimulation of gastric motility and emptying in diabetic gastroparesis. Ann Intern Med 1977;86:195–6.

42. Rao AS, Camilleri M. Review article: metoclopramide and tardive dyskinesia. Aliment Pharmacol Ther 2010;31:11–9.

43. Koch KL, Stern RM, Stewart WR, et al. Gastric emptying and gastric myoelectrical activity in patients with diabetic gastroparesis: effect of long-term domperidone treatment. Am J Gastroenterol 1989;84:1069–75.

44. Patterson D, Abell T, Rothstein R, et al. A double-blind multicenter comparison of domperidone and metoclopramide in the treatment of diabetic patients with symptoms of gastroparesis. Am J Gastroenterol 1999;94:1230–4.

45. Kessing BF, Smout AJ, Bennink RJ, et al. Prucalopride decreases esophageal acid exposure and accelerates gastric emptying in healthy subjects. Neurogastroenterol Motil 2014;26:1079–86.

46. Van Oudenhove L, Kindt S, Vos R, et al. Influence of buspirone on gastric sensorimotor function in man. Aliment Pharmacol Ther 2008;28:1326–33.

47. Tack J, Janssen P, Masaoka T, et al. Efficacy of buspirone, a fundus-relaxing drug, in patients with functional dyspepsia. Clin Gastroenterol Hepatol 2012;10: 1239–45.

48. Sawhney MS, Prakash C, Lustman PJ, et al. Tricyclic antidepressants for chronic vomiting in diabetic patients. Dig Dis Sci 2007;52:418–24.

49. Parkman HP, Van Natta ML, Abell TL, et al. Effect of nortriptyline on symptoms of idiopathic gastroparesis: the NORIG randomized clinical trial. JAMA 2013;310: 2640–9.

50. Malamood M, Roberts A, Kataria R, et al. Mirtazapine for symptom control in refractory gastroparesis. Drug Des Devel Ther 2017;11:1035–41.

51. Lin X, Liang J, Ren J, et al. Electrical stimulation of acupuncture points enhances gastric myoelectrical activity in humans. Am J Gastroenterol 1997;92:1527–30.

52. Wang CP, Kao CH, Chen WK, et al. A single-blinded, randomized pilot study evaluating effects of electroacupuncture in diabetic patients with symptoms suggestive of gastroparesis. J Altern Complement Med 2008;14:833–9.

53. Braden B, Caspary W, Börner N, et al. Clinical effects of STW 5 (Iberogast) are not based on acceleration of gastric emptying in patients with functional dyspepsia and gastroparesis. Neurogastroenterol Motil 2009;21:632–638,e5.

54. Miller LS, Szych GA, Kantor SB, et al. Treatment of idiopathic gastroparesis with injection of botulinum toxin into the pyloric sphincter muscle. Am J Gastroenterol 2002;97:1653–60.

55. Lacy BE, Zayat EN, Crowell MD, et al. Botulinum toxin for the treatment of gastroparesis: a preliminary report. Am J Gastroenterol 2002;97:1548–52.

56. Arts J, Holvoet L, Caenepeel P, et al. Clinical trial: a randomized-controlled cross-over study of intrapyloric injection of botulinum toxin in gastroparesis. Aliment Pharmacol Ther 2007;26:1251–8.
57. Friedenberg FK, Palit A, Parkman HP, et al. Botulinum toxin A for the treatment of delayed gastric emptying. Am J Gastroenterol 2008;103:416–23.
58. Coleski R, Anderson MA, Hasler WL. Factors associated with symptom response to pyloric injection of botulinum toxin in a large series of gastroparesis patients. Dig Dis Sci 2009;54:2634–42.
59. Clarke JO, Sharaiha RZ, Kord Valeshabad A, et al. Through-the-scope trans-pyloric stent placement improves symptoms and gastric emptying in patients with gastroparesis. Endoscopy 2013;45(Suppl 2 UCTN):E189–90.
60. Khashab MA, Besharati S, Ngamruengphong S, et al. Refractory gastroparesis can be successfully managed with endoscopic transpyloric stent placement and fixation (with video). Gastrointest Endosc 2015;82:1106–9.
61. Khashab MA, Stein E, Clarke JO, et al. Gastric peroral endoscopic myotomy for refractory gastroparesis: first human endoscopic pyloromyotomy (with video). Gastrointest Endosc 2013;78:764–8.
62. Mekaroonkamol P, Dacha S, Wang L, et al. Gastric peroral endoscopic pyloro-myotomy reduces symptoms, increases quality of life, and reduces health care use for patients with gastroparesis. Clin Gastroenterol Hepatol 2018. https://doi.org/10.1016/j.cgh.2018.04.016.
63. Khashab MA, Ngamruengphong S, Carr-Locke D, et al. Gastric per-oral endo-scopic myotomy for refractory gastroparesis: results from the first multicenter study on endoscopic pyloromyotomy (with video). Gastrointest Endosc 2017; 85:123–8.
64. Kahaleh M, Gonzalez JM, Xu MM, et al. Gastric peroral endoscopic myotomy for the treatment of refractory gastroparesis: a multicenter international experience. Endoscopy 2018. https://doi.org/10.1055/a-0596-7199.
65. Hibbard ML, Dunst CM, Swanström LL. Laparoscopic and endoscopic pyloro-plasty for gastroparesis results in sustained symptom improvement. J Gastrointest Surg 2011;15:1513–9.
66. Mancini SA, Angelo JL, Peckler Z, et al. Pyloroplasty for refractory gastroparesis. Am Surg 2015;81:738–46.
67. Shada AL, Dunst CM, Pescarus R, et al. Laparoscopic pyloroplasty is a safe and effective first-line surgical therapy for refractory gastroparesis. Surg Endosc 2016;30:1326–32.
68. Abell T, McCallum R, Hocking M, et al. Gastric electrical stimulation for medically refractory gastroparesis. Gastroenterology 2003;125:421–8.
69. McCallum RW, Snape W, Brody F, et al. Gastric electrical stimulation with Enterra therapy improves symptoms from diabetic gastroparesis in a prospective study. Clin Gastroenterol Hepatol 2010;8:947–54 [quiz: e116].
70. Daram SR, Tang SJ, Abell TL. Video: temporary gastric electrical stimulation for gastroparesis: endoscopic placement of electrodes (ENDOstim). Surg Endosc 2011;25:3444–5.
71. Jayanthi NV, Dexter SP, Sarela AI, et al. Gastric electrical stimulation for treatment of clinically severe gastroparesis. J Minim Access Surg 2013;9:163–7.
72. Fontana RJ, Barnett JL. Jejunostomy tube placement in refractory diabetic gas-troparesis: a retrospective review. Am J Gastroenterol 1996;91:2174–8.

Who Should Be Gluten-Free? A Review for the General Practitioner

Michelle Pearlman, MD, Lisa Casey, MD*

KEYWORDS

- Celiac disease • Wheat allergy • Nonceliac gluten sensitivity
- Nutritional deficiencies • Gastrointestinal symptoms

KEY POINTS

- A strict gluten-free diet is necessary in those with celiac disease and IgE-mediated wheat allergy.
- The prevalence of celiac disease is increasing and there are a significant number of individuals who remain undiagnosed.
- Following a gluten-free diet has become a popular fad diet in individuals who are trying to lose weight.
- Nonceliac gluten sensitivity is a poorly understood disorder in which patients have both intestinal and extraintestinal symptoms in response to gluten, although gluten exposure does not cause intestinal damage.
- Providers should understand how to evaluate for celiac disease and nonceliac gluten sensitivity and be aware of differences in the long-term risks and management options.

INTRODUCTION

Gluten is composed of a protein network that contributes to the elasticity and extensibility in bread and other commonly consumed products that contain wheat, rye, or barley.[1,2] Following a gluten-free diet (GFD) has become one of the most popular trends over the past decade. In a survey conducted by the National Restaurant Association in 2014, the GFD was voted 1 of the top 5 food trends. Gluten-free (GF) products may cost as much as 240% more than similar gluten-containing products,[3] and, despite this added cost, population surveys suggest that most of those endorsing a GFD do not have a formal diagnosis of celiac disease (CD).[4] Historically, GFDs were

Disclosure: There are no commercial or financial conflicts of interest. There are no funding sources for any of the authors.
Department of Internal Medicine, Division of Digestive and Liver Diseases, University of Texas Southwestern, 5323 Harry Hines Boulevard, Dallas, TX 75390-9151, USA
* Corresponding author.
E-mail address: Lisa.Casey@utsouthwestern.edu

Med Clin N Am 103 (2019) 89–99
https://doi.org/10.1016/j.mcna.2018.08.011
0025-7125/19/© 2018 Elsevier Inc. All rights reserved.

only recommended for those with a diagnosis of CD or IgE-mediated wheat allergy (WA), but more recently, as gluten-related disorders have come to the forefront of popular culture, people are following a GFD for numerous other reasons. As the number of GFD consumers increases, it is imperative that health care providers understand how to differentiate medical fact from popular fiction to effectively counsel their patients and limit potential complications.

Although a small percentage of individuals may be harmed by ingestion of particular foods due to food poisoning, food allergies, immune-mediated reasons, and food intolerances or sensitivities, food consumption is required for survival and benefits the vast majority of people. It is important to make a clear distinction among these various food-related entities because each one is associated with specific implications. Food poisoning, food allergy, and immune-mediated diseases cause significant complications and require strict avoidance, whereas intolerances and sensitivities result in less severe symptomology and thus do not require strict dietary avoidance. Beyond infectious etiologies, adverse food reactions are characterized as either immune mediated or non–immune mediated. Immune-mediated food reactions include those that are IgE mediated (hives and anaphylaxis), non–IgE mediated (food protein–induced enterocolitis syndrome and CD), cell mediated (allergic contact dermatitis), or mixed (eosinophilic esophagitis). Non–immune-mediated food reactions include metabolic (lactose intolerance and inborn errors of metabolism) and pharmacologic (reactivity to vasoactive amines in tyramine).[5] Approximately 1% of Americans have CD and 0.4% of Americans have WA. Based on the National Health and Nutrition Examination Survey diet study in 2009, which included 7798 persons, 0.63% followed a GFD although many of these individuals had neither CD nor WA.[4]

Not all gastrointestinal symptoms are considered true adverse food reactions. For example, it is physiologically normal to feel abdominal bloating after ingestion of a large meal, legumes, and/or cruciferous vegetables or high-fat foods because these foods enhance intestinal gas production or delay gastric emptying. Although these gastrointestinal symptoms may cause discomfort, none of these responses is considered pathologic.

CELIAC DISEASE: A HISTORICAL PERSPECTIVE

Wheat grain has been recognized as a human food source for thousands of years and has become a dietary staple in much of the world. Approximately one-third of the foods found in an American supermarket contain some component of wheat. Adverse symptoms attributed to gluten ingestion date as far back as the first century AD.[1] Despite the long hypothesized dietary link, it was not until the 1940s when Dutch physicians discovered that children with CD symptomatically improved when wheat and rye were scarce but subsequently deteriorated once bread was reintroduced into the diet by Allied forces.[6] A majority of American foods are regulated by the US Food and Drug Administration (FDA) but these exclude foods regulated by the US Department of Agriculture, such as meat, and also products, such as alcohol, tobacco, and cosmetics.

In 2004, the FDA Center for Food Safety and Applied Nutrition passed the 2004 Food Allergen Labeling and Consumer Protection Act, acknowledging the growing issue of food allergies and raising awareness. The FDA set goals for reporting on cross-contamination standards and GF labeling. Based on FDA standards, products may only be labeled GF if the product contains less than 20 parts per million of gluten.[7] This facilitated both awareness of food allergies and CD to the general public and aided patients with CD and WA in disease management.

The possibility that gluten might also cause problems in other individuals without CD was first suggested in a small case series of 8 patients with chronic diarrhea and abdominal pain in the 1980s. These patients experienced a dramatic relief on a GFD; however, symptoms returned when gluten was reintroduced. Small bowel biopsies of these patients were unremarkable and, as a result, this study raised questions regarding the role of gluten as a trigger for irritable bowel syndrome (IBS).[8] Given the wide overlap in nonspecific gastrointestinal symptoms between CD and IBS based on the Rome III criteria, many European countries began to recommend ruling out CD before diagnosing IBS.[9,10] More recently, there has been increased attention to the individuals who seem to have an intolerance to gluten and improve on a GFD but do not otherwise meet criteria for CD. These individuals have been noted to have both intraintestinal and extraintestinal symptoms. Although this disorder is still not well elucidated, it is currently known as nonceliac gluten sensitivity (NCGS).[11]

POP CULTURE: GOING GLUTEN-FREE

A major culture shift occurred with the publication of 2 best-selling self-help books, *Wheat Belly*, published by cardiologist William Davis, and *Grain Brain*, written by neurologist David Perlmutter. The vilification of wheat and gluten in these books seems to have created an empire founded on the premise that gluten is poison.[12] Both books were extremely successful because they reinforce powerful myths and promise simple dietary solutions to numerous health problems despite lack of sound evidence. The common theme in these books and others reiterates the importance of limiting processed foods and refined sugars and thus raises the question on whether it is gluten or actually alternate ingredients and/or chemicals found in processed foods that are the culprit for disease. Unfortunately, with much of the science taken out of context, these books and others can make it difficult to determine which individuals truly benefit from a GFD.

GLUTEN-RELATED DISORDERS: THE BASICS

CD is a non–IgE immune-mediated condition that is triggered by dietary gluten ingestion in genetically susceptible individuals. NCGS is a disorder in which patients develop both intraintestinal and extraintestinal symptoms after gluten exposure but do not meet criteria for CD or WA. WA is a hypersensitivity reaction to wheat proteins mediated via mast cell activation and immune mechanisms that are both IgE mediated and non–IgE mediated and affects between 0.5% and 4% of the population.[13] Additional diagnoses to consider in individuals who present with similar gastrointestinal symptoms include but are not limited to the following: NCGS, functional dyspepsia, eosinophilic gastroenteritis, IBS, inflammatory bowel disease, small intestinal bacterial overgrowth, connective tissue disorders, protein losing enteropathies (PLEs), common variable immune deficiency, microscopic colitis, and medication side effect.

CELIAC DISEASE: BASIC PRINCIPLES AND PATHOPHYSIOLOGY

The pathophysiology of CD is still not completely understood but is believed to result from a complex interplay among immunologic, genetic, and environmental factors. Ongoing research to study the pathophysiology of CD is essential to developing potential drug targets for treatment, particularly in those individuals who have refractory disease and do not respond to a strict GFD. Gluten is found in wheat, rye, barley, and crossbred hybrids of these 3 grains. Gluten is comprised of 2 peptides, glutenin and gliadin, which form a protein network and provide elasticity and extensibility in common food products and improve the texture and palatability. These peptides contain a high content of prolines and glutamines, which makes them resistant to degradation by gastric acid, pancreatic, and brush-border enzymes and allows them to remain in contact longer with mucosal surfaces and, in the setting of CD, cause intestinal damage.[6] In those with CD, gluten ingestion causes an immune response to gliadin in the intestinal lumen, which promotes an inflammatory reaction, primarily in the proximal small intestine. The inflammatory cascade is characterized by infiltration of the lamina propria and epithelium with chronic inflammatory cells and villous atrophy. The response is mediated by the innate and adaptive immune systems. Increased intestinal permeability allows transport of intact gliadin molecules through the small intestinal epithelium into the lamina propria where tissue transglutaminase (TTG) deamidates the gliadin peptides and increases their immunogenicity.[6]

CELIAC DISEASE: GENETIC FACTORS

CD has a strong genetic component. Epidemiologic studies report up to 20% of first-degree relatives are affected by the disease, with concordance rates of 75% to 80% with monozygotic twins and 10% in dizygotic twins. The best characterized genetic susceptibility factors are the HLA class II genes HLA-DQ2 and HLA-DQ8, which present antigens to immune cells. CD does not develop unless a person has alleles that encode for these proteins, although these alone are not sufficient to cause disease. The European Genetics Cluster on CD typed 1000 patients and found that 96% had either HLA-DQ2 or HLA-DQ8 genes. Although more advanced immunologic features of CD are beyond the scope of practice for most providers, these markers are believed to have an important role in screening because of their high negative predictive value. If a patient has obvious clinical disease in the setting of negative HLA-DQ2 or HLA-DQ8, however, this should not be ignored, given the potential for rare variants. The presence of these HLA gene variants changes geographically and may be used to assess CD risk and predict clinical course.[6,14–16]

CELIAC DISEASE: ENVIRONMENTAL FACTORS

The primary trigger in CD is exposure to gluten, which activates both adaptive and innate immune responses in the host gut epithelium. Studies suggest several environmental factors that may influence the development of CD and include timing of gluten introduction, cesarean delivery, lack of breast feeding, recurrent childhood gastrointestinal infections, and the host microbiome, although all of these factors continue to be under investigation.[17]

CELIAC DISEASE: SIGNS AND SYMPTOMS

Common presenting symptoms in children include vomiting, constipation, recurrent abdominal pain, growth issues, anemia, arthritis, neurologic symptoms, or no symptoms. In adults, symptoms at presentation vary widely and may include iron deficiency anemia, vitamin B_{12} deficiency, vitamin D deficiency, osteoporosis, bloating, heartburn, chronic fatigue, skin lesions, various neurologic and musculoskeletal presentations, and in some cases elevated liver enzymes and infertility (**Box 1**).[18]

CELIAC DISEASE: ASSOCIATED CONDITIONS

CD is often associated with other autoimmune conditions. Commonly associated conditions include but are not limited to autoimmune thyroid disease, dermatitis herpetiformis, recurrent oral aphthae, autoimmune liver and/or biliary disease, type 1

Box 1
Celiac disease: common signs and symptoms

Iron deficiency anemia

Vitamin D deficiency

Osteoporosis

Vitamin B_{12} deficiency

Bloating

Heartburn

Chronic fatigue

Skin rashes

Abnormal liver enzymes

Infertility

Vomiting

Diarrhea

Constipation

Recurrent abdominal pain

Growth problems

Arthritis

Neurologic symptoms

Asymptomatic

From Cronin CC, Shanahan F. Exploring the iceberg–the spectrum of celiac disease. Am J Gastroenterol 2003;98(3):518–20; with permission.

---

diabetes mellitus, Sjögren syndrome, Turner syndrome, Down syndrome, and Williams syndrome (**Box 2**).[19]

CELIAC DISEASE: SCREENING PRACTICES

CD for many years was believed a predominately pediatric disease characterized by diarrhea and malabsorption. Starting in the 1950s, major advancements were made in understanding the pathogenesis, diagnosis, and treatment of CD, including serologic testing and small bowel biopsy techniques. It is now clear that the disease spans all demographics and has a widely variable presentation.[20] Historically, individuals were only tested for CD when they presented with diarrhea and evidence of malabsorption; however, it seems that presenting symptoms vary and may depend on the region in which the patient resides. Advances in screening modalities in high-risk populations have increased diagnosis and identified a significant number of asymptomatic patients who previously would not have been screened.[21–25] Epidemiologic studies suggest that there are still large numbers of undiagnosed patients and also suggest the prevalence of CD is increasing for unclear reasons.[26–29]

CELIAC DISEASE: WHO TO SCREEN

The World Health Organization recommends mass screening for diseases that fulfill the following criteria: early clinical detection is difficult (diseases that have variable

---

Box 2
Celiac disease: common associated disorders

Autoimmune thyroid disease

Dermatitis herpetiformis

Recurrent oral aphthous ulcers

Autoimmune liver and/or biliary disease

Type 1 diabetes mellitus

Sjögren syndrome

Turner syndrome

Down syndrome

Williams syndrome

Modified from Rubio-Tapia A, Hill ID, Kelly CP, et al. ACG clinical guidelines: diagnosis and management of celiac disease. Am J Gastroenterol 2013;108(5):656–76; [quiz: 677]; with permission.

---

signs/symptoms or are asymptomatic); the condition affects at least 1% of the population; and available screening tests are highly sensitive and specific and effective treatments are available, whereas untreated disease can lead to complications. Some researchers argue that providers should perform universal screening because it is cost effective and can significantly increase a timely diagnosis, particularly given the myriad clinical manifestations and excessive health care utilization prior to diagnosis.[30,31] As such, there is a large volume of literature supporting more aggressive screening practices that may lead to a 40% increase in diagnosis.[26,28,32,33]

In traditional practice, screening for CD has been triggered by gastrointestinal symptoms of diarrhea or malabsorption. Increased knowledge of CD and heightened awareness of associated conditions have led to wider screening recommendations and include screening relatives and those with associated disorders (see **Box 2**). American College of Gastroenterology guidelines recommend screening individuals with signs or symptoms of malabsorption, laboratory evidence for CD, a first-degree relative with a diagnosis of CD even if the individual being tested is asymptomatic, elevated liver enzymes with no other clear etiology, and type 1 diabetes mellitus with signs/symptoms or laboratory evidence suggestive of CD.[19]

CELIAC DISEASE: DIAGNOSIS

A diagnosis of CD should be made based on blood tests and small intestinal biopsies. With the advent of serologic testing, TTG-IgA has a sensitivity and specificity of 95% with a greater likelihood of being a true positive result as the titer increases.[34,35] Given increased IgA deficiency in the celiac population, a normal IgA level should be confirmed. There is also a role for secondary serologies in some testing scenarios. Endomysial antibody is more costly, more subjective to interpretation, and less widely available, although highly sensitive, and can be useful in equivocal TTG testing scenarios. IgG deamidated gliadin can be useful in some scenarios, particularly in those patients who are IgA deficient.

Testing must be done on a gluten-containing diet, which has traditionally been a minimum of 10 g/d (approximately 4 slices of bread) for a period of 6 weeks, but more recent data suggest that possibly a smaller amount and a shorter interval are adequate in many cases. Greater than 3 g/d of gluten for 2 weeks has been demonstrated to produce histologic changes in 68% of patients.[36] Endoscopic biopsy remains the gold standard for confirmation of diagnosis.

A major limitation of the current diagnostic studies is that serologic testing and small bowel biopsies are only useful when an individual has current exposure to gluten. There is a high false-negative rate if testing is done while on a GFD, which reiterates the importance of early screening in high-risk or symptomatic individuals before they adopt a GFD. If individuals are already on a GFD, then they should be advised to reintroduce gluten prior to testing, if able. In practice, a large percentage of individuals are not willing to reintroduce gluten because of feeling poorly after re-exposure. In this circumstance, obtaining HLA-DQ2 and HLA-DQ8 can be helpful for ruling out a large proportion of individuals without CD if they do not have these alleles. Newer literature also suggests that an HLA-DQ gluten tetramer test might accurately identify or rule out patients with CD in the absence of gluten intake, although this is not yet widely accepted or available.[37]

CELIAC DISEASE TREATMENT

Treatment of those with CD is multidisciplinary and involves strict compliance with a GFD, education by a registered dietician, support groups to help with compliance, evaluation of bone health, and testing for/treating common micronutrient deficiencies.[19] To date, a strict GFD is the only accepted therapy for CD. Numerous alternate treatment modalities are under investigation, including enzyme therapies to digest gluten, polymers to bind gluten, probiotics, and therapies to alter permeability or tight junctions or to alter the immune or inflammatory response, including the use of vaccines to induce tolerance. Although studies are in progress, there are no new therapies approved to this point.[38]

Following a strict GFD has many challenges, although it has become easier over the past several decades because of increased availability and variety of GF foods. One of the major challenges for those who need to be strictly GF includes inadvertent gluten exposure from cross-contamination. Cross-contamination may occur when gluten-containing products are prepared in the same area as GF foods (cutting board, utensils, cookware, toaster, and storage containers) and from spreadable foods when utensils are used after contact with gluten-containing items. Practical tips for eating out include researching restaurants for GF items and/or calling ahead during off hours to talk to the chef directly about meal preparation.

Going GF does have some benefits. As discussed previously, following a GFD is necessary in those with IgE-mediated WA and CD, and, in CD, compliance improves intestinal healing and absorption of essential nutrients. Additional potential benefits of following a GFD that are inherent in following any strict nutrition plan include taking the time to read nutrition labels carefully, which may lead to decreased ingestion of many processed foods and refined sugars. Additionally, as the GFD trend grows in popularity, the availability and selection of GF foods have expanded and now include more palatable options and decreased risk of nutritional deficiencies, because more are being enriched with key vitamins and minerals, which they were previously devoid of.

DEBUNKING GLUTEN-FREE DIET MYTHS

The belief that GF products are "healthier" compared with similar gluten-containing products is not based on any sound evidence and in many cases is incorrect. GF products are commonly lower in fiber, iron, B vitamins, calcium, vitamin D, phosphorus, and zinc. Thompson and colleagues[39] illustrated that only 31% of women and 63%

of men who followed a GFD consumed recommended amounts of fiber, iron, and calcium. A 7-day prospective study comparing dietary intake patterns between 55 patients with CD on a GFD for greater than 2 years to 50 patients with newly diagnosed CD showed that more than 1 in 10 newly diagnosed and GFD-experienced women had inadequate intake of thiamine, folate, vitamin A, magnesium, calcium, and iron whereas more than 1 in 10 newly diagnosed men had inadequate thiamine, folate, magnesium, calcium, and zinc intake.[40] Furthermore, GF products commonly also contain more calories from fat and carbohydrates to improve palatability and texture because of the absence of gluten. Zuccotti and colleagues[41] compared macronutrient intake in 18 children with CD to 19 children without CD. The median energy intake in children with CD was significantly higher in calories, higher in carbohydrate intake, and lower in fat compared with healthy controls.

NONCELIAC GLUTEN SENSITIVITY

A large proportion of those individuals following a GFD are suggested to have NCGS. Although not well understood, NCGS does have a set of diagnostic criteria to help separate it from other gluten-related disorders based on a consensus meeting in 2015, called the Salerno criteria. NCGS is a clinical syndrome in which an individual describes intraintestinal and extraintestinal symptoms in response to ingestion of gluten and which improve in response to gluten avoidance, with CD and WA appropriately ruled out (including celiac serologies, small bowel biopsy as indicated, and wheat-specific IgE and skin prick test). The criteria suggest that optimally a double-blind, placebo-controlled gluten diet challenge containing 8 g/d of gluten without FODMAPs should be performed for confirmation but recognizes that this is not practical and, in most cases, not acceptable to patients.[11,42]

Although there have been reports that an older serology with low specificity for CD, IgG AGA, might be positive in some NCGS cases, there are no accepted serologies for diagnosis and no established genetic markers for diagnosis.[43] Compared with CD, with a prevalence of 1% and WA with a prevalence of 0.4%, NCGS is estimated to have a prevalence of between 0.63% and 6%.[44,45] Given the wide range of symptoms that cross over between other disorders, it is not clear if this prevalence truly represents NCGS or a range of disorders. The University of Maryland Center for Celiac Research performed a study between 2004 and 2010 of gluten-sensitive patients and reported the most common gluten-triggered symptoms included abdominal pain, eczema/rash, headache, difficulty focusing or foggy mind, fatigue, diarrhea, depression, anemia, numbness in the extremities, and joint pain.[45]

Studies of this patient population have suggested variable triggers, including gluten, FODMAP, wheat α-amylase/trypsin inhibitors, and perhaps even changes in the microbiome and dysbiosis.[46–49] The studies suggesting other sources of dietary trigger, such as FODMAPs, do not explain the extraintestinal symptoms that are common with this disorder. Further investigations are ongoing but this is currently accepted as a separate and unique gluten-related disorder.

SUMMARY

Unfortunately, awareness does not equal knowledge or understanding. Although there are clear medical indications for a GFD and clinical scenarios in which patients seem to symptomatically benefit from a GFD, there are also scenarios in which the risks of a GFD may outweigh benefit. Awareness of these differences facilitates appropriate diagnosis and counseling of patients and improves long-term management. With numerous ongoing studies of possible alternate CD treatments and investigations into the pathophysiology and diagnosis of NCGS, this is anticipated to be a continuously changing and robust field of study.

REFERENCES

1. Losowsky MS. A history of coeliac disease. Dig Dis 2008;26(2):112–20.
2. Wieser H. Chemistry of gluten proteins. Food Microbiol 2007;24(2):115–9.
3. Stevens L, Rashid M. Gluten-free and regular foods: a cost comparison. Can J Diet Pract Res 2008;69(3):147–50.
4. Rubio-Tapia A, Ludvigsson JF, Brantner TL, et al. The prevalence of celiac disease in the United States. Am J Gastroenterol 2012;107(10):1538–44 [quiz: 1537, 1545].
5. Boettcher E, Crowe SE. Dietary proteins and functional gastrointestinal disorders. Am J Gastroenterol 2013;108(5):728–36.
6. Kupfer SS, Jabri B. Pathophysiology of celiac disease. Gastrointest Endosc Clin N Am 2012;22(4):639–60.
7. Questions and answers: gluten- free food labeling final rule. 2017. Available at: https://www.fda.gov/Food/GuidanceRegulation/GuidanceDocumentsRegulatoryInformation/Allergens/ucm362880.htm. Accessed March 11, 2018.
8. Lundin KE, Alaedini A. Non-celiac gluten sensitivity. Gastrointest Endosc Clin N Am 2012;22(4):723–34.
9. Ford AC, Chey WD, Talley NJ, et al. Yield of diagnostic tests for celiac disease in individuals with symptoms suggestive of irritable bowel syndrome: systematic review and meta-analysis. Arch Intern Med 2009;169(7):651–8.
10. O'Leary C, Wieneke P, Buckley S, et al. Celiac disease and irritable bowel-type symptoms. Am J Gastroenterol 2002;97(6):1463–7.
11. Catassi C, Elli L, Bonaz B, et al. Diagnosis of Non-Celiac Gluten Sensitivity (NCGS): the salerno experts' Criteria. Nutrients 2015;7(6):4966–77.
12. Perlmutter DH. Grain brain: the surprising truth about wheat, carbs, and sugar–your brain's silent killers. Little, Brown and Company; 2013.
13. Hill ID, Fasano A, Guandalini S, et al. NASPGHAN clinical report on the diagnosis and treatment of gluten-related disorders. J Pediatr Gastroenterol Nutr 2016;63(1):156–65.
14. Megiorni F, Mora B, Bonamico M, et al. HLA-DQ and risk gradient for celiac disease. Hum Immunol 2009;70(1):55–9.
15. Megiorni F, Pizzuti A. HLA-DQA1 and HLA-DQB1 in Celiac disease predisposition: practical implications of the HLA molecular typing. J Biomed Sci 2012;19:88.
16. Karell K, Louka AS, Moodie SJ, et al. HLA types in celiac disease patients not carrying the DQA1*05-DQB1*02 (DQ2) heterodimer: results from the European Genetics Cluster on Celiac Disease. Hum Immunol 2003;64(4):469–77.
17. Stene LC, Honeyman MC, Hoffenberg EJ, et al. Rotavirus infection frequency and risk of celiac disease autoimmunity in early childhood: a longitudinal study. Am J Gastroenterol 2006;101(10):2333–40.
18. Farrell RJ, Kelly CP. Diagnosis of celiac sprue. Am J Gastroenterol 2001;96(12):3237–46.
19. Rubio-Tapia A, Hill ID, Kelly CP, et al. ACG clinical guidelines: diagnosis and management of celiac disease. Am J Gastroenterol 2013;108(5):656–76 [quiz: 677].
20. Cronin CC, Shanahan F. Exploring the iceberg–the spectrum of celiac disease. Am J Gastroenterol 2003;98(3):518–20.

21. Vivas S, Ruiz de Morales JM, Fernandez M, et al. Age-related clinical, serological, and histopathological features of celiac disease. Am J Gastroenterol 2008; 103(9):2360–5 [quiz: 2366].
22. Ludvigsson JF, Rubio-Tapia A, van Dyke CT, et al. Increasing incidence of celiac disease in a North American population. Am J Gastroenterol 2013;108(5):818–24.
23. Ludvigsson JF, Ansved P, Falth-Magnusson K, et al. Symptoms and signs have changed in Swedish children with coeliac disease. J Pediatr Gastroenterol Nutr 2004;38(2):181–6.
24. Reilly NR, Fasano A, Green PH. Presentation of celiac disease. Gastrointest Endosc Clin N Am 2012;22(4):613–21.
25. Reilly NR, Green PH. Epidemiology and clinical presentations of celiac disease. Semin Immunopathol 2012;34(4):473–8.
26. Fasano A, Berti I, Gerarduzzi T, et al. Prevalence of celiac disease in at-risk and not-at-risk groups in the United States: a large multicenter study. Arch Intern Med 2003;163(3):286–92.
27. Murray JA, Van Dyke C, Plevak MF, et al. Trends in the identification and clinical features of celiac disease in a North American community, 1950-2001. Clin Gastroenterol Hepatol 2003;1(1):19–27.
28. Catassi C, Kryszak D, Louis-Jacques O, et al. Detection of Celiac disease in primary care: a multicenter case-finding study in North America. Am J Gastroenterol 2007;102(7):1454–60.
29. Rubio-Tapia A, Kyle RA, Kaplan EL, et al. Increased prevalence and mortality in undiagnosed celiac disease. Gastroenterology 2009;137(1):88–93.
30. Green PH, Neugut AI, Naiyer AJ, et al. Economic benefits of increased diagnosis of celiac disease in a national managed care population in the United States. J Insur Med 2008;40(3–4):218–28.
31. Mattila E, Kurppa K, Ukkola A, et al. Burden of illness and use of health care services before and after celiac disease diagnosis in children. J Pediatr Gastroenterol Nutr 2013;57(1):53–6.
32. Katz KD, Rashtak S, Lahr BD, et al. Screening for celiac disease in a North American population: sequential serology and gastrointestinal symptoms. Am J Gastroenterol 2011;106(7):1333–9.
33. Green PH. Where are all those patients with Celiac disease? Am J Gastroenterol 2007;102(7):1461–3.
34. Lewis NR, Scott BB. Meta-analysis: deamidated gliadin peptide antibody and tissue transglutaminase antibody compared as screening tests for coeliac disease. Aliment Pharmacol Ther 2010;31(1):73–81.
35. van der Windt DA, Jellema P, Mulder CJ, et al. Diagnostic testing for celiac disease among patients with abdominal symptoms: a systematic review. JAMA 2010;303(17):1738–46.
36. Lebwohl B, Sanders DS, Green PHR. Coeliac disease. Lancet 2018;391(10115): 70–81.
37. Sarna VK, Lundin KEA, Morkrid L, et al. HLA-DQ-Gluten tetramer blood test accurately identifies patients with and without celiac disease in absence of gluten consumption. Gastroenterology 2018;154(4):886–96.e6.
38. Haridy J, Lewis D, Newnham ED. Investigational drug therapies for coeliac disease - where to from here? Expert Opin Investig Drugs 2018;27(3):225–33.
39. Thompson T, Dennis M, Higgins LA, et al. Gluten-free diet survey: are Americans with coeliac disease consuming recommended amounts of fibre, iron, calcium and grain foods? J Hum Nutr Diet 2005;18(3):163–9.

40. Shepherd SJ, Gibson PR. Nutritional inadequacies of the gluten-free diet in both recently-diagnosed and long-term patients with coeliac disease. J Hum Nutr Diet 2013;26(4):349–58.
41. Zuccotti G, Fabiano V, Dilillo D, et al. Intakes of nutrients in Italian children with celiac disease and the role of commercially available gluten-free products. J Hum Nutr Diet 2013;26(5):436–44.
42. Igbinedion SO, Ansari J, Vasikaran A, et al. Non-celiac gluten sensitivity: all wheat attack is not celiac. World J Gastroenterol 2017;23(40):7201–10.
43. Carroccio A, Mansueto P, Iacono G, et al. Non-celiac wheat sensitivity diagnosed by double-blind placebo-controlled challenge: exploring a new clinical entity. Am J Gastroenterol 2012;107(12):1898–906 [quiz: 1907].
44. Fasano A, Sapone A, Zevallos V, et al. Nonceliac gluten sensitivity. Gastroenterology 2015;148(6):1195–204.
45. Sapone A, Bai JC, Ciacci C, et al. Spectrum of gluten-related disorders: consensus on new nomenclature and classification. BMC Med 2012;10:13.
46. Biesiekierski JR, Newnham ED, Irving PM, et al. Gluten causes gastrointestinal symptoms in subjects without celiac disease: a double-blind randomized placebo-controlled trial. Am J Gastroenterol 2011;106(3):508–14 [quiz: 515].
47. Biesiekierski JR, Peters SL, Newnham ED, et al. No effects of gluten in patients with self-reported non-celiac gluten sensitivity after dietary reduction of fermentable, poorly absorbed, short-chain carbohydrates. Gastroenterology 2013; 145(2):320–8.e1-3.
48. Biesiekierski JR, Muir JG, Gibson PR. Is gluten a cause of gastrointestinal symptoms in people without celiac disease? Curr Allergy Asthma Rep 2013;13(6): 631–8.
49. Junker Y, Zeissig S, Kim SJ, et al. Wheat amylase trypsin inhibitors drive intestinal inflammation via activation of toll-like receptor 4. J Exp Med 2012;209(13): 2395–408.

Diet and the Role of Food in Common Gastrointestinal Diseases

Michelle Pearlman, MD[a],*, Oviea Akpotaire, MD[b]

KEYWORDS

- Artificial sweeteners • Dairy • Lactose intolerance • Fiber • Diverticulosis
- Hepatic encephalopathy • Protein

KEY POINTS

- The use of artificial sweeteners as sugar substitutes is not an optimal tool for weight loss.
- Most individuals with self-reported lactose intolerance do not have objective lactose malabsorption.
- Most individuals with lactose intolerance can tolerate up to 12 g of lactose and complete dairy avoidance should be minimized.
- High-fiber diets do not prevent the formation of diverticula but are generally recommended to decrease the risk of symptomatic diverticular disease.
- Cirrhotic patients benefit from high-protein diets to help with malnutrition and sarcopenia. Dietary protein consumption does not seem to contribute to worsening hepatic encephalopathy.

INTRODUCTION

Nutrition plays an essential role in normal cellular processes and is required for survival of all living organisms. Food, however, can also be perceived as a necessary evil in select individuals who have food allergies, intolerances, and certain diseases. This article focuses particularly on the role of food in common gastrointestinal and liver diseases and debunks popular dietary myths.

Disclosure Statement: There are no commercial or financial conflicts of interest. There are no funding sources for any of the authors.
[a] Gastroenterology and Hepatology Fellow, Department of Internal Medicine, Division of Digestive and Liver Diseases, University of Texas Southwestern, 5323 Harry Hines Boulevard, Dallas, TX 75390-9151, USA; [b] Department of Internal Medicine, University of Texas Southwestern, 5323 Harry Hines Boulevard, Dallas, TX 75390-9151, USA
* Corresponding author.
E-mail address: m.pearlman@med.miami.edu

Med Clin N Am 103 (2019) 101–110
https://doi.org/10.1016/j.mcna.2018.08.008
0025-7125/19/© 2018 Elsevier Inc. All rights reserved.

medical.theclinics.com

THE USE OF ARTIFICIAL SWEETENERS AS A WEIGHT LOSS TOOL
Obesity Risk Factors

Obesity is a major public health problem that has become increasingly more prevalent over the last several decades.[1] Studies suggest that obesity is a consequence of numerous internal host factors and environmental factors, including genetics, consumption of energy-rich foods that are predominantly high in fat and sugar, physical inactivity, and alterations in the host microbiome.[2–5]

The Evolution of Artificial Sweetener and Overcompensation

Artificial sweetener (AS) was originally developed as a sugar substitute based on the premise that using these products in place of sugar would lead to decreased caloric intake, improve insulin resistance, and ultimately result in weight loss.[6–8] AS is low in calories and are either not metabolized by the host or activate sweet taste receptors at such small quantities that the calories associated with the AS are negligible. Despite the intended and theoretic benefits of AS, there are a significant amount of data to suggest that AS consumption has a negative impact on the host microbiome, gut-brain axis, glucose homeostasis, energy consumption, and body adiposity. The addition of AS to otherwise unsweetened foods or liquids improves palatability and promotes increased caloric consumption in both animals and humans.[8,9] One study compared calorie consumption in participants given either diet beverages or water. Participants drinking diet beverages consumed less dessert but the overall caloric intake remained similar between the 2 groups.[10] Similar findings were demonstrated by Tey and colleagues[11] in 30 healthy men. Despite saving calories with a diet beverage compared with a sucrose-containing beverage, participants who consumed a diet beverage before an ad libitum lunch had similar daily caloric intake because of overcompensation during subsequent meals. In another study, 8 obese participants who were aware they were consuming aspartame-containing products ingested similar or slightly more calories compared with participants given a conventional diet without AS. When the diet was covertly changed from the conventional diet to the aspartame-containing diet, participants had a 25% spontaneous reduction in caloric intake, suggesting that part of the increased caloric consumption attributed to AS is based on a conscious or subconscious decision to eat more.[12] As these studies have shown, despite the premise that AS should promote weight loss, it does not seem to reduce overall caloric intake.

The Effects of Artificial Sweetener on Body Weight

Numerous studies have demonstrated a positive association between AS and increased body mass index (BMI) in a dose-dependent fashion.[13–15] In 2033 healthy mothers, Azad and colleagues[16] demonstrated that maternal consumption of artificially sweetened beverages during pregnancy was associated with a greater infant BMI and a 2-fold higher risk of being overweight at 1 year of age. Additionally, a meta-analysis showed a pooled relative risk (RR) of obesity of 1.18 in participants who consumed sugar-containing soda compared with an RR of 1.59 in those who consumed diet soda.[17] Long-term use of AS is also associated with weight gain, as illustrated in a cohort study of 1454 participants with a median follow-up of 10 years. In this study, participants consuming AS had a significantly increased BMI and waist circumference compared with AS nonusers.[18] In summary, despite marketing claims that suggest AS are a better alternative to sugar, research studies suggest that AS are not an adequate tool to aid in weight loss.

LACTOSE INTOLERANCE
Lactose Intolerance: Basic Principles

Dairy products contain important macronutrients, such as protein and fat, and are the principal source of calcium in most diets.[19] Lactose is the main carbohydrate source in milk products and lactose powder is used in many foods. The lactase enzyme is located in the small intestine and hydrolyzes lactose to glucose and galactose.[20] In patients with lactose intolerance, lactose is not adequately digested and absorbed in the small intestine, leading to fermentation by colonic bacteria and intestinal gas production. Multiple variables influence lactose tolerance, including age, gender, genetics, host lactase activity, the lactose load, and concurrent food ingestion. Other factors influencing lactose tolerance include the rate of gastric emptying, duration of contact with the small bowel mucosa, ability of the colonic flora to ferment unabsorbed lactose, and sensitivity of the small bowel and colon to distention as intestinal fluid secretion occurs in response to the osmotic load from unabsorbed lactose.[21] Individuals with lactose intolerance frequently report nausea, abdominal pain, bloating, and diarrhea.[22] Many patients who complain of these symptoms either choose to avoid dairy on their own or are advised by their health care providers to do so. Despite these common practices, symptom improvement after a trial of dairy avoidance has not been shown to correlate with whether a person has true lactose malabsorption.

Lactose Intolerance and Dairy Avoidance: A Review of the Evidence

Lactase deficiency is the most frequent cause for malabsorption and affects greater than 65% of the world's adult population.[23,24] Half-levels of lactase activity are sufficient to digest 50 g of lactose, which is the amount used in the standard lactose tolerance test. A hydrogen (H_2) breath test is considered positive when there is an elevation of breath H_2 greater than 20 ppm following ingestion of 50 g of lactose.[25] Most individuals with lactose intolerance can tolerate up to 12 g of lactose or about 1 cup of milk without significant symptoms.[26,27]

The National Institutes of Health Consensus Conference on Lactose Intolerance and Health concluded that most people with lactose malabsorption do not have clinical lactose intolerance and patients who self-report lactose intolerance may not truly be lactose malabsorbers. In 2011, the Australian Bureau of Statistics performed a cross-sectional survey of 1184 adults and found that 17% reported dairy avoidance due to an allergy or intolerance, although most lacked a formal diagnosis.[28] Yang and colleagues[25] studied the effects of lactose ingestion on individuals with irritable bowel syndrome-diarrhea (IBS-D). Sixty participants with IBS-D and 60 controls underwent H_2 breath testing to detect lactose malabsorption after ingestion of varying lactose doses. The study showed that lactose malabsorption was associated with higher doses of lactose ingestion in both groups and was not more frequent in participants with IBS-D. Despite the similar rates of lactose malabsorption, participants with IBS-D self-reported lactose intolerance more frequently than controls, and self-reported lactose intolerance did not correlate with a positive H_2 breath test. Casellas and colleagues[23] conducted a 3-year, prospective, cross-sectional study of 580 participants referred for H_2 breath testing and examined lactose malabsorption, self-reported lactose intolerance, and quality of life. The study showed that 56% of study participants self-reported lactose intolerance, which was associated with dairy avoidance and lower health-related quality of life scores compared with participants with objective lactose malabsorption that was not clearly associated with dairy avoidance. This finding suggests self-perception of lactose intolerance affects the decision to avoid dairy more than true lactose malabsorption.

Lactose Intolerance and the Microbiome

In those with lactose malabsorption, colonic bacteria ferment the undigested lactose, which leads to gas production. As such, the host microbiome may influence the degree of lactose intolerance because some colonic bacteria can use undigested sugars compared with other bacteria that ferment them. There are some data to suggest that regular dairy consumption in patients with lactase deficiency may lead to colonic adaptation by the host microbiome by increasing fecal beta-galactosidase activity; that is, lactose-fermenting organisms that do not produce H_2.[29]

Complications of Dairy Avoidance

Because many individuals with nonspecific gastrointestinal symptoms either choose to avoid or are advised to avoid all dairy products, they have an increased risk of metabolic bone disease and fractures from inadequate calcium consumption, and an increased risk of metabolic syndrome.[19,30–32]

There are several strategies to minimize symptoms related to lactose ingestion while maximizing calcium and vitamin D intake. These include eating small amounts of lactose at a time by consuming low-lactose products (eg, yogurt or hard cheeses), taking lactose-digesting products (eg, beta-galactosidase enzyme) before dairy consumption, and taking calcium and vitamin D supplements dietary if intake is inadequate.[33–35] Finally, it is important to develop educational programs and behavioral approaches for patients and health care providers to minimize potential complications resulting from complete dairy avoidance and to help improve symptoms in patients with nonspecific gastrointestinal symptoms that may or may not be related to true lactose malabsorption.[36]

DIVERTICULAR DISEASE
Classification and Epidemiology of Diverticular Disease

Diverticular disease (DD) is typically asymptomatic and incidentally discovered during colonoscopy or imaging. Of patients with diverticula, about 25% have clinical symptoms that range from alterations in bowel patterns to bleeding or diverticulitis.[37] Diverticulitis can be further categorized as uncomplicated (inflammation of 1 of more diverticula) versus complicated, which is when abscess, perforation, fistula formation, or obstruction occur.[38] The prevalence of DD increases with age. It affects less than 10% of patients aged younger 40 years, 33% by age 60 years, and up to 50% to 70% by age 80 years.[37,39–41]

Diverticular Disease: Discovery and Pathophysiology

The development of DD is influenced by age, genetics, diet, colonic microbiota, colonic motility, and colonic structure; however, the underlying mechanisms remain unclear.[42] DD was first described in late 1800s in patients who underwent surgery for peritonitis, and the association between constipation and acute diverticulitis was recognized soon after. Low-fiber diets were initially preferred in patients with DD to prevent food fragments from getting lodged in the diverticula because this was thought to be a nidus for inflammation and infection. In the 1970s, however, Painter and Burkitt[40] noted that the incidence of deaths related to DD increased 10-fold to 15-fold in developed countries. They hypothesized that the low-fiber, high-fat Western diet was the culprit. They also theorized that prolonged stool transit time caused a functional obstruction, increasing intraluminal pressure and producing the mucosal outpouchings known as diverticula.

Diverticular Disease: The Role of Fiber and Avoidance of Nuts and Seeds

Over time, common practice has shifted toward recommending high-fiber diets to decrease stool transit time; however, there is a paucity of data to support this theory.[37]

One meta-analysis of 19 studies examined the effect of fiber intake on symptomatic, uncomplicated DD and found only low-quality evidence to suggest a possible benefit.[43] Another meta-analysis of 8 studies of participants with acute uncomplicated diverticulitis found low quality of evidence to suggest that a high-fiber diet results in a decreased risk of diverticulitis recurrence and/or symptomatic DD. Despite low-quality evidence, the investigators concluded that participants with DD should still consume a high-fiber diet because the potential overall health benefits outweigh the risks. The investigators also recommend a liberalized diet following an episode of acute diverticulitis because no evidence was found to support specific dietary restrictions.[44] In another study of 264 nonvegetarians and 56 vegetarians, fiber intake and the presence of DD on imaging was examined. On contrast enema studies, 33% of nonvegetarians and 13% of vegetarians had diverticulosis and vegetarians consumed more fiber than nonvegetarians (42 g/d vs 21 g/d). However, vegetarians with diverticula consumed more fiber (34 g/d) than nonvegetarians without diverticula (22 g/d), and the nonvegetarians with and without diverticulosis consumed similar amounts of fiber. These findings suggest that additional risk factors contribute to the development of diverticula regardless of fiber intake or type of diet.[45]

Several very large studies have also examined fiber intake and DD. In a large study of 44,000 men between the ages of 40 to 75 years without prior DD, Aldoori and colleagues[46] compared the highest (>32 g/d) versus lowest quintiles of dietary fiber intake and found that insoluble fiber consumption was associated with a decreased risk of developing symptomatic DD. A subsequent study in 46,000 men found an increased risk of diverticulitis associated with a Western diet after adjusting for fiber intake.[41] The European Prospective Investigation into Cancer and Nutrition (EPIC) prospective cohort study of 47,000 participants showed a decreased risk of hospital admissions for diverticulitis in participants who consumed high-fiber diets (>25 g/d) versus less than 14 g per day.[47] Finally, in 690,075 middle-aged women, higher dietary fiber intake was associated with a decreased risk of DD and varied based on fiber source.[48]

Studies that evaluate the role of fiber in DD have several limitations, including the accuracy of dietary recall questionnaires, using subjective gastrointestinal symptoms to assess for symptomatic DD, and making positive or negative associations based on case-control or cross-sectional studies that do not assess lifelong dietary habits.[39] Currently, the data suggest that adequate dietary fiber intake may reduce risk of complications in those with DD.

Despite lack of supporting evidence, individuals with DD have been advised to avoid nuts and seeds that could theoretically become lodged in diverticula and result in diverticulitis.[38,39,46,49] One study evaluated the association between nut, corn, and popcorn consumption and risk of diverticulitis and diverticular bleeding in 47,228 adult men. During the 18-year follow up period, there was actually an inverse association between nut and popcorn consumption and risk of diverticulitis, and no association with diverticular bleeding.[50] It is unnecessary to counsel patients with DD to avoid nuts, seeds, and popcorn. Instead, patients should be encouraged to consume a healthy diet with adequate fiber intake.

HEPATIC ENCEPHALOPATHY
Hepatic Encephalopathy and Protein Consumption

Among the frequently encountered complications of cirrhosis, the genesis of hepatic encephalopathy (HE) remains only partially understood.[51] A normal liver can convert ammonia to urea for renal excretion; however, liver dysfunction from advanced fibrosis or portosystemic shunting can lead to ureagenesis and precipitate HE.[51,52] The prevalence of protein-calorie malnutrition in cirrhotic patients ranges from 40% to 70%, worsens with disease severity, and negatively affects mortality even following liver transplantation.[53–57] This effect is accentuated when cirrhotic patients are advised to limit dietary protein intake to reduce ammonia production and theoretically reduce the risk of HE.

The Pathophysiology of Malnutrition and Sarcopenia in Cirrhosis

Liver fibrosis prevents adequate glycogen storage, reduces glycogenolysis, triggers catabolism of muscle and fat for gluconeogenesis and ketogenesis, and ultimately leads to sarcopenia and adipopenia.[54,56–62] To further complicate the problem, decompensated cirrhotic patients tend to have low oral intake in the setting of symptomatic ascites and may also have a degree of malabsorption and/or maldigestion from portal enteropathy or in the setting of cholestasis.[56,59,63–66] Performing an accurate nutritional assessment of patients with severe liver dysfunction is often quite difficult, especially in the setting of ascites and poor synthetic function. Interestingly, malnutrition and sarcopenia may be associated with HE at the molecular level and have been shown to be independent risk factors for overt HE in several studies.[58,67] Increased myocyte ammonia concentration induces skeletal muscle autophagy, suggesting that impaired ammonia clearance may worsen sarcopenia. Conversely, decreased muscle mass prevents myocyte conversion of ammonia to glutamine for renal excretion, suggesting that sarcopenia may also enhance HE.[68] Additionally, digestion of dietary protein generates aromatic amino acids (AAAs) and branched-chain amino acids (BCAAs). Muscle tissue uses BCAAs but not AAAs for myocyte protein synthesis because muscle only contains branched-chain keto-dehydrogenase. Cirrhotic patients have depleted serum BCAA concentrations and increased serum AAA concentrations, which further promotes adaptive muscle autophagy and sarcopenia.[52,54,69]

Dietary Protein Intake in Cirrhosis

Research suggests that, in addition to alcohol cessation, exercise, adequate micronutrient supplementation, and utilization of lactulose and rifaximin, consuming dietary protein with frequent meals is beneficial in limiting the degree of malnutrition and the risk of HE.[51,54,70] The European Society for Clinical Nutrition (ESPEN) recommends 1.2 to 1.5 g/kg per day of protein before and after liver transplant, and enteral BCAA supplementation.[71] One review of 9 randomized controlled trials (RCTs) of cirrhotic adults favored BCAA therapy over other nutritional supplements for the treatment of HE, with similar findings reported in a Cochrane review of 16 RCTs.[72,73] It is also recommended that cirrhotic patients consume protein from a variety of sources, including dairy (casein), plants that are rich in BCAAs, and animal protein.[54,74] Although it is generally recommended that cirrhotic patients consume high-protein diets, a study found that limiting protein intake for 3 days following transjugular intrahepatic portosystemic shunt placement and then progressively increasing protein consumption significantly reduced the occurrence of HE.[75]

FUTURE CONSIDERATIONS AND SUMMARY

Patients follow certain dietary practices for gastrointestinal and liver symptoms and diseases that are often not supported by scientific evidence and rely mainly on popular beliefs. These include use of AS for weight loss, which has been contradicted by several research studies showing no loss of weight with AS use, and avoiding nuts and seeds to avoid symptomatic DD, although high-fiber diets may have a protective effect in patients with diverticula. Appropriate counseling for patients with possible lactose intolerance and patients with cirrhosis at risk for HE is important. Finally, educational programs are needed for internists, subspecialists, and other medical professionals to improve patient education and minimize potential complications that can occur as a result of restrictive dietary practices.

REFERENCES

1. Sturm R, Hattori A. Morbid obesity rates continue to rise rapidly in the United States. Int J Obes (Lond) 2013;37(6):889–91.
2. De Filippo C, Cavalieri D, Di Paola M, et al. Impact of diet in shaping gut microbiota revealed by a comparative study in children from Europe and rural Africa. Proc Natl Acad Sci U S A 2010;107(33):14691–6.
3. Mbakwa CA, Scheres L, Penders J, et al. Early life antibiotic exposure and weight development in children. J Pediatr 2016;176:105–13.e102.
4. Panduro A, Rivera-Iniguez I, Sepulveda-Villegas M, et al. Genes, emotions and gut microbiota: the next frontier for the gastroenterologist. World J Gastroenterol 2017;23(17):3030–42.
5. Segata N. Gut microbiome: westernization and the disappearance of intestinal diversity. Curr Biol 2015;25(14):R611–3.
6. Ponce CH, Brown MS, Silva JS, et al. Effects of a dietary sweetener on growth performance and health of stressed beef calves and on diet digestibility and plasma and urinary metabolite concentrations of healthy calves. J Anim Sci 2014;92(4):1630–8.
7. Shearer J, Swithers SE. Artificial sweeteners and metabolic dysregulation: lessons learned from agriculture and the laboratory. Rev Endocr Metab Disord 2016;17(2):179–86.
8. Sterk A, Schlegel P, Mul AJ, et al. Effects of sweeteners on individual feed intake characteristics and performance in group-housed weanling pigs. J Anim Sci 2008;86(11):2990–7.
9. Benton D. Can artificial sweeteners help control body weight and prevent obesity? Nutr Res Rev 2005;18(1):63–76.
10. Piernas C, Tate DF, Wang X, et al. Does diet-beverage intake affect dietary consumption patterns? Results from the Choose Healthy Options Consciously Everyday (CHOICE) randomized clinical trial. Am J Clin Nutr 2013;97(3): 604–11.
11. Tey SL, Salleh NB, Henry J, et al. Effects of aspartame-, monk fruit-, Stevia-, and sucrose-sweetened beverages on postprandial glucose, insulin and energy intake. Int J Obes (Lond) 2017;41(3):450–7.
12. Porikos KP, Booth G, Van Itallie TB. Effect of covert nutritive dilution on the spontaneous food intake of obese individuals: a pilot study. Am J Clin Nutr 1977; 30(10):1638–44.
13. Colditz GA, Willett WC, Stampfer MJ, et al. Patterns of weight change and their relation to diet in a cohort of healthy women. Am J Clin Nutr 1990;51(6):1100–5.

14. Fowler SP, Williams K, Resendez RG, et al. Fueling the obesity epidemic? Artificially sweetened beverage use and long-term weight gain. Obesity (Silver Spring) 2008;16(8):1894–900.
15. Stellman SD, Garfinkel L. Artificial sweetener use and one-year weight change among women. Prev Med 1986;15(2):195–202.
16. Azad MB, Sharma AK, de Souza RJ, et al. Association between artificially sweetened beverage consumption during pregnancy and infant body mass index. JAMA Pediatr 2016;170(7):662–70.
17. Ruanpeng D, Thongprayoon C, Cheungpasitporn W, et al. Sugar and artificially-sweetened beverages linked to obesity: a systematic review and meta-analysis. QJM 2017;110(8):513–20.
18. Chia CW, Shardell M, Tanaka T, et al. Chronic low-calorie sweetener use and risk of abdominal obesity among older adults: a cohort study. PLoS One 2016;11(11): e0167241.
19. Weaver CM. Should dairy be recommended as part of a healthy vegetarian diet? Point. Am J Clin Nutr 2009;89(5):1634S–7S.
20. Bayless TM, Brown E, Paige DM. Lactase non-persistence and lactose intolerance. Curr Gastroenterol Rep 2017;19(5):23.
21. Bedine MS, Bayless TM. Intolerance of small amounts of lactose by individuals with low lactase levels. Gastroenterology 1973;65(5):735–43.
22. Lomer MC, Parkes GC, Sanderson JD. Review article: lactose intolerance in clinical practice–myths and realities. Aliment Pharmacol Ther 2008;27(2):93–103.
23. Casellas F, Aparici A, Perez MJ, et al. Perception of lactose intolerance impairs health-related quality of life. Eur J Clin Nutr 2016;70(9):1068–72.
24. Szilagyi A. Adult lactose digestion status and effects on disease. Can J Gastroenterol Hepatol 2015;29(3):149–56.
25. Yang J, Deng Y, Chu H, et al. Prevalence and presentation of lactose intolerance and effects on dairy product intake in healthy subjects and patients with irritable bowel syndrome. Clin Gastroenterol Hepatol 2013;11(3):262–8.e1.
26. Argnani F, Di Camillo M, Marinaro V, et al. Hydrogen breath test for the diagnosis of lactose intolerance, is the routine sugar load the best one? World J Gastroenterol 2008;14(40):6204–7.
27. Shaukat A, Levitt MD, Taylor BC, et al. Systematic review: effective management strategies for lactose intolerance. Ann Intern Med 2010;152(12):797–803.
28. Statistics ABo. Australian health survey: nutrition first results- food and nutrients, 2011-12. 2011-2012. Available at: http://www.abs.gov.au/ausstats/abs@.nsf/mf/4364.0.55.007. Accessed April 29, 2018.
29. Levitt M, Wilt T, Shaukat A. Clinical implications of lactose malabsorption versus lactose intolerance. J Clin Gastroenterol 2013;47(6):471–80.
30. Appleby P, Roddam A, Allen N, et al. Comparative fracture risk in vegetarians and nonvegetarians in EPIC-Oxford. Eur J Clin Nutr 2007;61(12):1400–6.
31. Carroccio A, Montalto G, Cavera G, et al. Lactose intolerance and self-reported milk intolerance: relationship with lactose maldigestion and nutrient intake. Lactase Deficiency Study Group. J Am Coll Nutr 1998;17(6):631–6.
32. Szilagyi A, Galiatsatos P, Xue X. Systematic review and meta-analysis of lactose digestion, its impact on intolerance and nutritional effects of dairy food restriction in inflammatory bowel diseases. Nutr J 2016;15(1):67.
33. Brown-Riggs C. Nutrition and health disparities: the role of dairy in improving minority health outcomes. Int J Environ Res Public Health 2015;13(1). ijerph13010028.

34. Opstelten JL, Leenders M, Dik VK, et al. Dairy products, dietary calcium, and risk of inflammatory bowel disease: results from a European prospective cohort investigation. Inflamm Bowel Dis 2016;22(6):1403–11.

35. Paige DM, Bayless TM, Graham GG. Pregnancy and lactose intolerance. Am J Clin Nutr 1973;26(3):238–40.

36. Suchy FJ, Brannon PM, Carpenter TO, et al. National institutes of health consensus development conference: lactose intolerance and health. Ann Intern Med 2010;152(12):792–6.

37. Aldoori W, Ryan-Harshman M. Preventing diverticular disease. Review of recent evidence on high-fibre diets. Can Fam Physician 2002;48:1632–7.

38. Rezapour M, Ali S, Stollman N. Diverticular disease: an update on pathogenesis and management. Gut Liver 2018;12(2):125–32.

39. Bohm SK. Risk factors for diverticulosis, diverticulitis, diverticular perforation, and bleeding: a plea for more subtle history taking. Viszeralmedizin 2015;31(2): 84–94.

40. Painter NS, Burkitt DP. Diverticular disease of the colon: a deficiency disease of Western civilization. Br Med J 1971;2(5759):450–4.

41. Strate LL, Keeley BR, Cao Y, et al. Western dietary pattern increases, and prudent dietary pattern decreases, risk of incident diverticulitis in a prospective cohort study. Gastroenterology 2017;152(5):1023–30.e1022.

42. Tursi A. Dietary pattern and colonic diverticulosis. Curr Opin Clin Nutr Metab Care 2017;20(5):409–13.

43. Carabotti M, Annibale B, Severi C, et al. Role of fiber in symptomatic uncomplicated diverticular disease: a systematic review. Nutrients 2017;9(2) [pii:E161].

44. Dahl C, Crichton M, Jenkins J, et al. Evidence for dietary fibre modification in the recovery and prevention of reoccurrence of acute, uncomplicated diverticulitis: a systematic literature review. Nutrients 2018;10(2) [pii:E137].

45. Gear JS, Ware A, Fursdon P, et al. Symptomless diverticular disease and intake of dietary fibre. Lancet 1979;1(8115):511–4.

46. Aldoori WH, Giovannucci EL, Rockett HR, et al. A prospective study of dietary fiber types and symptomatic diverticular disease in men. J Nutr 1998;128(4): 714–9.

47. Crowe FL, Appleby PN, Allen NE, et al. Diet and risk of diverticular disease in Oxford cohort of European Prospective Investigation into Cancer and Nutrition (EPIC): prospective study of British vegetarians and non-vegetarians. BMJ 2011;343:d4131.

48. Crowe FL, Balkwill A, Cairns BJ, et al. Source of dietary fibre and diverticular disease incidence: a prospective study of UK women. Gut 2014;63(9):1450–6.

49. Schechter S, Mulvey J, Eisenstat TE. Management of uncomplicated acute diverticulitis: results of a survey. Dis Colon Rectum 1999;42(4):470–5 [discussion: 475–6].

50. Strate LL, Liu YL, Syngal S, et al. Nut, corn, and popcorn consumption and the incidence of diverticular disease. JAMA 2008;300(8):907–14.

51. Chadalavada R, Sappati Biyyani RS, Maxwell J, et al. Nutrition in hepatic encephalopathy. Nutr Clin Pract 2010;25(3):257–64.

52. Campollo O, Sprengers D, Dam G, et al. Protein tolerance to standard and high protein meals in patients with liver cirrhosis. World J Hepatol 2017;9(14):667–76.

53. Alberino F, Gatta A, Amodio P, et al. Nutrition and survival in patients with liver cirrhosis. Nutrition 2001;17(6):445–50.

54. Anand AC. Nutrition and muscle in cirrhosis. J Clin Exp Hepatol 2017;7(4): 340–57.

55. Englesbe MJ, Patel SP, He K, et al. Sarcopenia and mortality after liver transplantation. J Am Coll Surg 2010;211(2):271–8.
56. Plauth M, Schutz ET. Cachexia in liver cirrhosis. Int J Cardiol 2002;85(1):83–7.
57. Tsien CD, McCullough AJ, Dasarathy S. Late evening snack: exploiting a period of anabolic opportunity in cirrhosis. J Gastroenterol Hepatol 2012;27(3):430–41.
58. Kalaitzakis E, Olsson R, Henfridsson P, et al. Malnutrition and diabetes mellitus are related to hepatic encephalopathy in patients with liver cirrhosis. Liver Int 2007;27(9):1194–201.
59. Peng S, Plank LD, McCall JL, et al. Body composition, muscle function, and energy expenditure in patients with liver cirrhosis: a comprehensive study. Am J Clin Nutr 2007;85(5):1257–66.
60. Petrides AS, DeFronzo RA. Glucose and insulin metabolism in cirrhosis. J Hepatol 1989;8(1):107–14.
61. Owen OE, Reichle FA, Mozzoli MA, et al. Hepatic, gut, and renal substrate flux rates in patients with hepatic cirrhosis. J Clin Invest 1981;68(1):240–52.
62. Owen OE, Trapp VE, Reichard GA Jr, et al. Nature and quantity of fuels consumed in patients with alcoholic cirrhosis. J Clin Invest 1983;72(5):1821–32.
63. Ferreira LG, Ferreira Martins AI, Cunha CE, et al. Negative energy balance secondary to inadequate dietary intake of patients on the waiting list for liver transplantation. Nutrition 2013;29(10):1252–8.
64. Shanbhogue RL, Bistrian BR, Jenkins RL, et al. Resting energy expenditure in patients with end-stage liver disease and in normal population. JPEN J Parenter enteral Nutr 1987;11(3):305–8.
65. Stamoulis I, Kouraklis G, Theocharis S. Zinc and the liver: an active interaction. Dig Dis Sci 2007;52(7):1595–612.
66. Charlton M. Energy and protein metabolism in alcoholic liver disease. Clin Liver Dis 1998;2:781–98.
67. Merli M, Giusto M, Lucidi C, et al. Muscle depletion increases the risk of overt and minimal hepatic encephalopathy: results of a prospective study. Metab Brain Dis 2013;28(2):281–4.
68. Brown R. New advances in hepatic encephalopathy, vol. 19. Elsevier; 2015.
69. Dasarathy S, Merli M. Sarcopenia from mechanism to diagnosis and treatment in liver disease. J Hepatol 2016;65(6):1232–44.
70. Amodio P, Bemeur C, Butterworth R, et al. The nutritional management of hepatic encephalopathy in patients with cirrhosis: international society for hepatic encephalopathy and nitrogen metabolism consensus. Hepatology 2013;58(1):325–36.
71. Plauth M, Cabre E, Riggio O, et al. ESPEN guidelines on enteral nutrition: liver disease. Clin Nutr 2006;25(2):285–94.
72. Metcalfe EL, Avenell A, Fraser A. Branched-chain amino acid supplementation in adults with cirrhosis and porto-systemic encephalopathy: systematic review. Clin Nutr 2014;33(6):958–65.
73. Gluud LL, Dam G, Les I, et al. Branched-chain amino acids for people with hepatic encephalopathy. Cochrane Database Syst Rev 2017;(5):CD001939.
74. Dasarathy S. Nutrition and alcoholic liver disease: effects of alcoholism on nutrition, effects of nutrition on alcoholic liver disease, and nutritional therapies for alcoholic liver disease. Clin Liver Dis 2016;20(3):535–50.
75. Luo L, Fu S, Zhang Y, et al. Early diet intervention to reduce the incidence of hepatic encephalopathy in cirrhosis patients: post-Transjugular Intrahepatic Portosystemic Shunt (TIPS) findings. Asia Pac J Clin Nutr 2016;25(3):497–503.

Colorectal Cancer Screening
Is Colonoscopy the Best Option?

Peter S. Liang, MD, MPH[a,b], Jason A. Dominitz, MD, MHS[c,d],*

KEYWORDS

- Colorectal cancer • Screening • Colonoscopy • Fecal immunochemical test
- Fecal occult blood test • Sigmoidoscopy • Guidelines • Effectiveness

KEY POINTS

- Screening for colorectal cancer, the second leading cause of cancer death in the United States, is effective for reducing cancer incidence and mortality.
- Of the available screening tests, fecal occult blood testing, flexible sigmoidoscopy, and colonoscopy have the most robust evidence of benefit.
- The quality of colonoscopy has been found to be highly variable across providers, and this variability is associated with cancer mortality and incidence.
- Randomized controlled trials comparing colonoscopy and fecal immunochemical testing are ongoing and will provide definitive data for comparative effectiveness.
- Providers should consider effectiveness, safety, patient preference, and cost when deciding which screening test to recommend.

INTRODUCTION

Colorectal cancer (CRC) is the second most common cancer in women and the third most common in men worldwide.[1] In the United States, CRC is the second leading cause of cancer death among men and women (estimated 50,630 deaths in 2018), with a lifetime incidence of 1 in 22 in men and 1 in 24 in women. However, CRC incidence and mortality have been decreasing over the past several decades.[2] Screening

Disclosure: The authors have no relevant financial disclosures.

This material is the result of work supported in part by resources from The Veterans Health Administration. The views expressed in this article are those of the authors and do not represent the views of the Department of Veterans Affairs.

[a] Gastroenterology Section, Department of Medicine, VA New York Harbor Health Care System, 423 East 23rd Street, 11N, New York, NY 10010, USA; [b] Division of Gastroenterology, Department of Medicine, NYU Langone Health, New York, NY, USA; [c] Gastroenterology Section, VA Puget Sound Health Care System, 1660 South Columbian Way, Seattle, WA 98108, USA; [d] Division of Gastroenterology, Department of Medicine, University of Washington School of Medicine, Seattle, WA, USA

* Corresponding author. VA Puget Sound Health Care System, 1660 South Columbian Way, Seattle, WA 98108.

E-mail address: Jason.Dominitz@va.gov

accounts for half of the reduction in incidence and mortality,[3] which is accomplished by removing precancerous polyps and detecting early stage cancer.[4]

CRC is the only cancer for which screening has been proven to reduce mortality for average-risk women and men. Randomized controlled trials (RCTs) for guaiac-based fecal occult blood test (gFOBT) and flexible sigmoidoscopy, and observational studies for colonoscopy, demonstrate these three screening tests all significantly reduce CRC mortality. In addition, four large RCTs are currently studying the effect of screening colonoscopy on CRC mortality.[5–8] Despite the robust evidence supporting screening, uptake in the general population is suboptimal. In 2015, only 62% of Americans aged 50 to 75 were up to date on screening.[9] Because an estimated 46% to 63% of CRC deaths are attributable to nonscreening, efforts to increase screening adherence are of paramount importance.[10]

Although the availability of screening options may boost adherence through providing individuals with choice based on personal preferences, it may also lead to confusion among providers as to which screening test to recommend, and among patients as to what screening to undergo. This article provides an overview of the available test options and the evidence for each; a summary of major guidelines; and a comparison of the two most widely used tests, colonoscopy and fecal immunochemical testing (FIT).

DESCRIPTION AND EVIDENCE FOR VARIOUS COLORECTAL CANCER SCREENING TESTS
Noninvasive Tests

Guaiac fecal occult blood test
gFOBT detects the presence of blood in stool through the pseudoperoxidase activity of heme, a breakdown product of blood hemoglobin, in stool samples that are self-collected by the patient and sent to the laboratory. Five RCTs with long-term follow-up (11–30 years) have shown that compared with no screening, biennial gFOBT reduced CRC mortality by 9% to 22%.[11–15] One trial compared either annual or biennial gFOBT with usual care and found that annual screening resulted in greater mortality reduction (32% vs 22%) through 30 years of follow-up.[15] This Minnesota-based study was also the only trial that found a reduction in CRC incidence (20% for annual and 17% for biennial gFOBT) compared with usual care.[16] Of note, these trials used an older gFOBT with lower sensitivity for CRC than the high-sensitivity gFOBTs that are currently available. For high-sensitivity gFOBTs, sensitivity for CRC ranges from 62% to 79% and specificity ranges from 87% to 96%.[17,18] Limitations of gFOBT include the need to avoid certain medications (eg, nonsteroidal anti-inflammatory drugs), foods (eg, meat, fish, and some raw vegetables), and vitamin C because of the potential for false-positive or false-negative results.[19] Also, adherence with screening is challenging because of the recommendation for testing three stool samples annually.

Fecal immunochemical test
FIT has emerged as a preferred test over gFOBT because of several advantages. Although FIT also tests self-collected stool samples, it relies on an immunochemical test for antibodies to the globin component of human hemoglobin. Therefore, no dietary modification is required. Most FITs only require one stool sample, and comparative studies have demonstrated superior adherence with FIT over gFOBT.[20] A meta-analysis found the pooled sensitivity and specificity of FIT for CRC was 79% and 94%, respectively.[21] Although there are no RCTs that demonstrate CRC mortality reduction using FIT, it is widely considered the preferred screening test for fecal occult blood

because of its greater sensitivity for CRC than gFOBT and the previously mentioned logistical advantages. Screening with FIT may be most effective within the context of an organized screening program (ie, programmatic screening) in order to ensure high-quality screening processes.[22,23]

Fecal immunochemical test DNA

The multitarget stool DNA test combines a FIT with testing for molecular markers of abnormal DNA. Individuals mail a whole stool sample along with a separate FIT kit directly to the manufacturer, who also provides an integrated patient navigation process with the test to improve adherence. In a large trial comparing FIT-DNA with FIT in average-risk adults who underwent colonoscopy, FIT-DNA was more sensitive (92% vs 74%) but less specific (87% vs 95%) than FIT for CRC.[23] FIT-DNA was also more sensitive for the detection of sessile serrated polyps measuring greater than or equal to 10 mm (42.4% vs 5.1%). The programmatic sensitivity and specificity of FIT-DNA (which is currently recommended every 3 years) compared with annual FIT screening is unknown, but a cost-effectiveness analysis suggests FIT is more effective and less costly than FIT-DNA under most plausible scenarios.[24]

Computed tomography colonography

Computed tomography (CT) colonography generally involves a bowel preparation followed by a CT scan with insufflation of the colon via a rectal balloon catheter. Digital 3-dimensional renderings of the colon allow for a virtual "fly through" of the colon to look for polyps or other lesions (**Fig. 1**). CT colonography studies have used adenomas greater than or equal to 6 or 10 mm, rather than CRC, as the outcome to measure performance characteristics. The pooled sensitivity for adenomas greater than or equal to 10 mm is 89%, whereas the specificity is 94%. For adenomas greater than or equal to 6 mm, the pooled sensitivity and specificity are 86% and 88%, respectively.[25] Concerns about CT colonography relate to its radiation dose, incidental extracolonic findings, and limited detection of serrated lesions.[26]

Capsule colonoscopy

Capsule colonoscopy requires a large-volume bowel preparation similar to colonoscopy, ingestion of a pill-sized camera that records images throughout the colon, and additional booster doses of laxative or prokinetic medications to propel the capsule into the colon. The procedure is not approved by the US Food and Drug Administration as a first-line screening test, but it is approved for patients in whom colonoscopy was technically unsuccessful and for those with evidence of lower gastrointestinal bleeding and at high risk for colonoscopy or moderate sedation. The sensitivity and specificity of capsule colonoscopy is 92% and 95% for adenomas greater than or equal to 10 mm and 88% and 82% for adenomas greater than or equal to 6 mm.[27] As with CT colonography, however, serrated lesions are not well detected by capsule colonoscopy.

Septin9

The only blood-based screening test currently approved by the Food and Drug Administration detects methylated septin9 DNA, which is associated with CRC. However, this test is only approved for patients who have declined screening tests that are recommended by the 2008 US Preventive Services Task Force (USPSTF) guidelines, including high-sensitivity gFOBT, FIT, colonoscopy, and flexible sigmoidoscopy. In a trial that studied an older version of the test, the age-standardized sensitivity and specificity for CRC were 48% and 92%, respectively.[28] The currently approved version of the test has a sensitivity for CRC of 68% and specificity of 79%.[29]

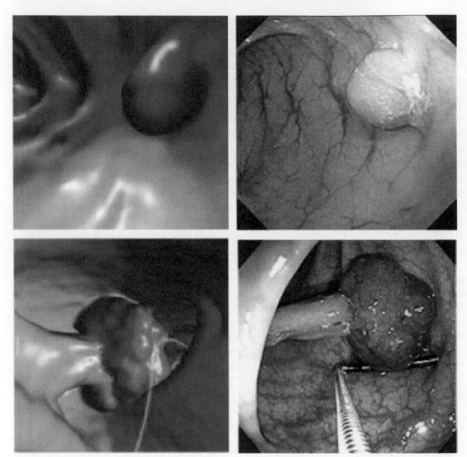

Fig. 1. Polyps seen on CT colonography versus colonoscopy. CT colonography images (*left*) and corresponding colonoscopic views (*right*). (*Courtesy of* B.D. Cash, MD, Houston, TX.)

Invasive Tests

Colonoscopy

Colonoscopy is the only screening test that can visualize and remove precancerous polyps from the entire colon, and it is the recommended diagnostic test when any of the other screening tests detects an abnormality. Colonoscopy requires dietary modification and a bowel preparation, and it is usually performed with sedation. Currently, data from clinical trials evaluating the effectiveness of colonoscopy on CRC incidence and mortality are unavailable. However, the proven CRC mortality and incidence benefits seen in RCTs of gFOBT are believed to result from diagnostic colonoscopies (often with polypectomy) performed in response to positive gFOBT. Moreover, in addition to retrospective studies showing an association between colonoscopy and improved CRC outcomes,[30,31] one large prospective cohort study with 22 years of follow-up found screening colonoscopy was associated with a 68% reduction in CRC mortality and a 43% to 56% reduction in CRC incidence.[32]

The benefits of colonoscopy have been shown to be highly operator-dependent. In a study of 135 gastroenterologists practicing in a large integrated health care system in California, each 1% increase in the gastroenterologists' adenoma detection rate was associated with a 3% reduction in the incidence of CRC after colonoscopy and a 5% reduction in CRC mortality.[33] As a result of this and other studies, increasing attention has been paid to the importance of ensuring high-quality colonoscopy.[34] For practices where programmatic CRC screening is challenging, colonoscopy may be a preferred approach because of the longer interval between tests.

Flexible sigmoidoscopy

Flexible sigmoidoscopy enables direct visualization and biopsy and/or removal of polyps from the distal half of the colon. Unlike colonoscopy, no sedation is required and enemas usually suffice for bowel preparation. Four RCTs with long-term follow-up (11–17 years) have evaluated flexible sigmoidoscopy compared with no screening.[35–38] A meta-analysis of these trials showed that flexible sigmoidoscopy reduced CRC mortality by 27% (18%–34%) and reduced CRC incidence by 21% (15%–25%).[25] The data show that women benefit less from flexible sigmoidoscopy than men, although the magnitude of the difference is inconsistent across trials.

Table 1 summarizes the comparative characteristics of the previously discussed screening tests.

SUMMARY OF MAJOR GUIDELINES
US Preventive Services Task Force

The Affordable Care Act stipulates that preventive services that carry an "A" or "B" recommendation from the USPSTF must be covered by all insurers. Because USPSTF recommendations directly dictate national health policy, it is often considered the gold standard. The most recent 2016 USPSTF recommendation on CRC screening[39] was a considerable departure from the previous 2008 version, where the USPSTF gave an "A" recommendation to screening adults aged 50 to 75 with high-sensitivity FOBT annually, flexible sigmoidoscopy every 5 years with high-sensitivity FOBT every 3 years, and colonoscopy every 10 years. In the 2016 update, CRC screening in general is given an "A" recommendation for the 50 to 75 age group. The USPSTF chose to list available screening test options (**Table 2**), and stated that they "found no head-to-head studies demonstrating that any of the screening strategies [they] considered are more effective than others, although the tests have varying levels of evidence supporting their effectiveness, as well as different strengths and limitations." Therefore, rather than presenting test options in a preferred or ranked order, they suggested that offering a choice in strategies may increase adherence and have the largest impact on CRC outcomes.

US Multi-Society Task Force on Colorectal Cancer

The US Multi-Society Task Force on Colorectal Cancer (MSTF) represents the three national gastroenterology societies in the United States: the American College of Gastroenterology, the American Gastroenterological Association, and the American Society for Gastrointestinal Endoscopy. In contrast to the USPSTF recommendation, the 2017 MSTF recommendations ranked screening tests in tiers based on performance features, costs, and practical considerations.[40] FIT and colonoscopy were considered the only Tier 1 options (see **Table 2**). Additionally, the MSTF outlined three strategies for providers to offer screening in a nonprogrammatic (ie, opportunistic) setting: (1) providing individuals with multiple choices at the beginning, (2) offering one test at a time in a sequential approach, or (3) risk-stratifying individuals based on demographic and medical factors and recommending colonoscopy for those at high risk versus noninvasive testing for those at low risk.

Table 1
Comparative characteristics of colorectal cancer screening tests

Test	Evidence of Efficacy	Home-Based Screening	Bowel Preparation	Invasiveness	Sedation	Other
Colonoscopy	Prospective cohort study: 68% lower mortality[32] Retrospective studies show reduced mortality and incidence		++	+++	+	Allows removal of polyps at time of examination
FIT	No mortality data 79% sens, 94% spec for CRC[21]	+		[a]		
gFOBT	RCT: 32% lower mortality, 20% lower incidence with annual screening[15,16]	+		[a]		
Flexible sigmoidoscopy	RCT: 27% (18%–34%) lower mortality, 21% (15%–25%) lower incidence[25]		+	++[a]		Declining availability because of limited reimbursement
Flexible sigmoidoscopy + FIT	RCT: 38% lower mortality[56]		+	++[a]		Declining availability because of limited reimbursement
CT colonography	No mortality data 86% (78%–95%) sens, 88% (82%–94%) spec for adenomas ≥6 mm[25]		++	+[a]		Variable availability because of reimbursement and expertise; concerns about extracolonic findings and radiation exposure
FIT-DNA	No mortality data 92% sens, 87% spec for CRC[23]	+		[a]		Uncertainty about appropriate surveillance interval
Septin9 DNA	No mortality data 68% sens, 79% spec for CRC[29]			[a]		Not approved as first-line test; variable availability because of reimbursement; limited experience; uncertainty about appropriate testing interval
Capsule colonoscopy	No mortality data 88% sens, 82% spec for adenomas ≥6 mm[27]		+++	+[a]		Not approved as first-line test; variable availability because of reimbursement; concerns about technical failure rate, need for more bowel preparation than colonoscopy

Abbreviations: sens, sensitivity; spec, specificity.
[a] Requires diagnostic colonoscopy if screening test is positive.

Table 2
Summary of colorectal cancer screening guidelines

Test	USPSTF (2016) Frequency Between Testing (y)	Ranking	MSTF (2017) Frequency Between Testing (y)	Ranking	CTFPHC (2016) Frequency Between Testing (y)	Ranking
Colonoscopy	10	None	10	Tier 1	—	NR
FIT	1		1	Tier 1	2	R
gFOBT	1		—		2	R
Flexible sigmoidoscopy	5		10 (or 5)	Tier 2	10	R
Flexible sigmoidoscopy + FIT	10 + 1		—	—	—	—
CT colonography	5		5	Tier 2	—	—
FIT-DNA	1 or 3		3	Tier 2	—	—
Septin9 DNA	—		—	NR	—	—
Capsule colonoscopy	—		5	Tier 3	—	—

Abbreviations: CTFPHC, Canadian Task Force on Preventive Health Care; MSTF, Multi-Society Task Force; NR, not recommended; R, recommended; USPSTF, US Preventive Services Task Force.

Canadian Task Force on Preventive Health Care

Compared with guidelines from US organizations, the Canadian Task Force on Preventive Health Care recommendations discuss fewer tests options and only recommend gFOBT, FIT, and flexible sigmoidoscopy (see **Table 2**).[41] Notably, colonoscopy is not recommended because of the absence of RCT evidence supporting a mortality reduction, the need for greater human resources (ie, trained endoscopists), and a greater potential for harms.

Putting Guidelines into Context

The three guidelines previously highlighted were chosen to illustrate the spectrum of organizational perspective with respect to CRC screening. It is not a comprehensive list, because other primary care, gastroenterology, oncology, and radiology organizations have published their own recommendations. The USPSTF chose not to rank the test options to offer a greater choice of screening tests, with the goal of increasing population-level screening rates. However, this approach has been criticized because it effectively placed tests with and without evidence for CRC mortality reduction on equal footing. On the other end of the spectrum, the Canadian Task Force on Preventive Health Care focused only on RCT evidence and therefore excluded many of the test options considered by the USPSTF and MSTF. It also included an accompanying cost-effectiveness analysis,[42] which is important for policy and implementation but generally absent from US guidelines. The MSTF recommendation acknowledged varying levels of evidence supporting different screening tests, but it also considered practical issues of test availability and reimbursement in its tiered approach. Therefore, flexible sigmoidoscopy, which has RCT evidence for mortality reduction but is no longer widely used in clinical practice, is presented as a Tier 2 option along with FIT-DNA and CT colonography. Practitioners who work within an organization often need to operate under institutional guidelines that define the available screening tests. For health care organizations and individual practitioners, understanding the rationale behind these guidelines enables a more informed decision about which screening tests to offer to patients and in what order to do so.

UNCERTAINTY: COLONOSCOPY VERSUS FECAL IMMUNOCHEMICAL TEST

Fecal occult blood testing (gFOBT and FIT) is the most widely used screening modality worldwide. In contrast, colonoscopy is the predominant screening test in the United States, where only 11% of individuals who were up to date with screening reported that they had received a stool-based test.[43] Because the controversy surrounding the best screening test centers around colonoscopy versus FIT, we compare several aspects of these two modalities in the following section.

Effectiveness

To date, there is no RCT data on the effectiveness of either FIT or colonoscopy or their comparative effectiveness for preventing CRC or mortality. Four RCTs currently being conducted in Europe and the United States will provide definitive and complementary evidence for the effectiveness of these modalities (**Table 3**).[5–8] The CONFIRM study,[6] which is being conducted at 46 Veterans Affairs medical centers, is comparing colonoscopy with annual FIT, whereas the Spanish COLONPREV trial is comparing colonoscopy and biennial FIT.[5] Baseline results of the COLONPREV study reveal similar rates of CRC detection after one round of FIT screening, although colonoscopy did find more advanced neoplasia. It remains to be seen how future FIT screening rounds will impact cancer outcomes. The Swedish SCREESCO study has three arms[8] (colonoscopy, two rounds of FIT in Years 1 and 3, and no screening), whereas the multinational NordICC trial is comparing colonoscopy with no screening.[7] However, because these are all long-term CRC mortality studies, the earliest results are not expected until approximately 2021.

Screening with FIT is recommended every 1 to 2 years, compared with every 10 years for colonoscopy, and long-term adherence to multiple rounds of testing is thought to be crucial for the effectiveness of the FIT strategy. Data have shown that adherence to FOBT declines rapidly over time in clinical practice,[44] but how this affects CRC outcomes is unknown. Comparing results from the SCREESCO, COLONPREV, and CONFIRM trials, which respectively entail 2, 5, and 10 rounds of FIT, will demonstrate whether the quantity and frequency of testing impacts effectiveness.

Cost-Effectiveness

Existing cost-effectiveness analyses consistently demonstrate that FIT and colonoscopy are cost-effective or cost-saving compared with no screening.[45] A modeling

Table 3
Randomized controlled trials of colonoscopy and FIT effectiveness

Study	Country	Age	Enrollment	Arms	Primary Outcome
CONFIRM[6]	United States	50–75	50,000	Colonoscopy vs annual FIT	10-y CRC mortality
COLONPREV[5]	Spain	50–69	57,404	Colonoscopy vs biennial FIT	10-y CRC mortality
NordICC[7]	Poland Norway Netherlands Sweden	55–64	94,959	Colonoscopy vs no screening	15-y CRC mortality
SCREESCO[8]	Sweden	59–62	200,000	Colonoscopy vs FIT (in Years 1 and 3) vs no screening	15-y CRC mortality

study conducted to inform the 2016 USPSTF guidelines showed that screening the 50 to 75 age group with colonoscopy every 10 years would require a median 15 colonoscopies per life-year gained, compared with seven colonoscopies per life-year gained using annual FIT.[46]

Complications

Major complications of colonoscopy include cardiopulmonary events, gastrointestinal bleeding, and perforation. In a meta-analysis of population-based studies, the pooled prevalence for perforation, postcolonoscopy bleeding, and mortality were 0.5/1000, 2.6/1000, and 2.9/100,000 colonoscopies.[47] Because patients who have a positive FIT are recommended to undergo a diagnostic colonoscopy, the complication rate is directly related to the number of lifetime colonoscopies that are performed in each screening strategy. It is estimated that for every 1000 people aged 50 to 75, screening with colonoscopy every 10 years would result in a median 4049 colonoscopies and 15 complications, compared with 1757 colonoscopies and 10 complications for annual FIT.[46]

Other Considerations

Several other aspects of colonoscopy and FIT deserve mention. First, although colonoscopy is touted as a screening test that is only needed every 10 years, this interval is recommended for those with no neoplastic polyps (eg, adenomas). However, adenomas are found in more than 25% of screening colonoscopies, leading to surveillance recommendations of 3 to 5 years for many individuals.[34] Also, endoscopists frequently recommend shorter surveillance intervals than the guidelines recommend. It has been shown that 46% of individuals with a negative colonoscopy receive a repeat procedure within 7 years.[48] Colonoscopy overuse is widespread and has important implications for patient safety and health care costs, but unfortunately it is not considered in formal analyses of cost and harm.

Second, although 25% of colonoscopies in the United States are performed for surveillance of polyps,[49] there is currently no evidence that surveillance reduces CRC incidence or mortality. Guidelines recommend that patients with low-risk adenomas (<3 adenomas, <10 mm in size, no high-risk histologic features) undergo surveillance colonoscopy in 5 to 10 years,[50] but most endoscopists recommend a 5-year follow-up.[51] However, data suggest such frequent surveillance may be unnecessary. In a recent study with a median follow-up of 13 years, individuals with adenomas less than 10 mm and without high-risk histologic features at baseline colonoscopy had no increased risk of CRC incidence or mortality compared with those with no adenomas.[52] In contrast, individuals with adenomas greater than or equal to 10 mm or with high-risk histologic features had a 2.7-fold higher risk of CRC incidence and 2.6-fold higher risk of mortality. The EPoS I study, an RCT being conducted in Europe, will compare CRC incidence in patients with low-risk adenomas who are randomized to surveillance colonoscopy at 5 and 10 years or 10 years only.[53] Findings from this trial are not expected until 2028 but will provide important data for more evidence-based and cost-effective surveillance guidelines.

Third, any noncolonoscopic screening test that is positive should be evaluated with a diagnostic colonoscopy. However, many studies have documented poor adherence with this evaluation and a delay of 10 months has been shown to increase CRC risk.[22,54] Quality assurance systems should be put into place to facilitate adherence with every step in the screening process (eg, completion of FIT kits, notification of results, timely referral for diagnostic colonoscopy, appropriate rescreening or surveillance).[22]

Finally, providers who are considering whether to offer colonoscopy or FIT, or any other screening test, should adopt the shared decision-making approach and solicit patient preference. Some individuals prefer an invasive test with high sensitivity and the opportunity to remove polyps at the time of screening, despite the inconvenience and risk. Others prefer the convenience of screening at home, despite the need for more frequent testing. Not only is shared decision-making consistent with the principle of patient-centered care, but data also show that giving patients a choice of two testing options can improve screening rates.[55]

FUTURE CONSIDERATIONS/SUMMARY

Screening has been proven to reduce CRC incidence and prevent deaths from this common and deadly disease. Of the various screening options available, FOBT, flexible sigmoidoscopy, and colonoscopy possess the most robust evidence of benefit. However, the predominant tests used today are FIT and colonoscopy, and trials comparing their effectiveness are underway. Currently, there is no clear-cut "best" test for CRC screening. Whether or not colonoscopy is ultimately determined to be the "best" test, it is clearly the test of choice for the evaluation of patients found to have a positive screening test (eg, FIT). But the effectiveness of colonoscopy is highly dependent on various operator characteristics, highlighting the importance of ongoing quality assurance efforts. Until the results are in from the ongoing clinical trials of screening colonoscopy, health care providers should focus on improving adherence to screening and make recommendations to their patients that take into account considerations of effectiveness, safety, patient preference, and cost.

ACKNOWLEDGMENTS

The authors thank Douglas Robertson, MD, MPH, for his comments on an earlier version of this article.

REFERENCES

1. Ferlay J, Soerjomataram I, Ervik M, et al. GLOBOCAN 2012 v1.0, cancer incidence and mortality worldwide: IARC CancerBase No. 11. Lyon (France): International Agency for Research on Cancer; 2013. Available at: http://globocan.iarc.fr. Accessed May 4, 2018.
2. Siegel RL, Miller KD, Jemal A. Cancer statistics, 2018. CA Cancer J Clin 2018; 68(1):7–30.
3. Edwards BK, Ward E, Kohler BA, et al. Annual report to the nation on the status of cancer, 1975-2006, featuring colorectal cancer trends and impact of interventions (risk factors, screening, and treatment) to reduce future rates. Cancer 2010; 116(3):544–73.
4. Zauber AG, Winawer SJ, O'Brien MJ, et al. Colonoscopic polypectomy and long-term prevention of colorectal-cancer deaths. N Engl J Med 2012;366(8):687–96.
5. Quintero E, Castells A, Bujanda L, et al. Colonoscopy versus fecal immunochemical testing in colorectal-cancer screening. N Engl J Med 2012;366(8):697–706.
6. Dominitz JA, Robertson DJ, Ahnen DJ, et al. Colonoscopy vs. fecal immunochemical test in reducing mortality from colorectal cancer (CONFIRM): rationale for study design. Am J Gastroenterol 2017;112(11):1736–46.
7. Bretthauer M, Kaminski MF, Løberg M, et al. Population-based colonoscopy screening for colorectal cancer: a randomized clinical trial. JAMA Intern Med 2016;176(7):894–902.

8. SCREESCO - Screening of Swedish colons. Available at: https://clinicaltrials.gov/ct2/show/NCT02078804. Accessed May 4, 2018.

9. White A, Thompson TD, White MC, et al. Cancer screening test use—United States, 2015. MMWR Morb Mortal Wkly Rep 2017;66(8):201–6.

10. Meester RGS, Doubeni CA, Lansdorp-Vogelaar I, et al. Colorectal cancer deaths attributable to nonuse of screening in the United States. Ann Epidemiol 2015; 25(3):208–13.e1.

11. Faivre J, Dancourt V, Lejeune C, et al. Reduction in colorectal cancer mortality by fecal occult blood screening in a French controlled study. Gastroenterology 2004; 126(7):1674–80.

12. Kronborg O, Jørgensen OD, Fenger C, et al. Randomized study of biennial screening with a faecal occult blood test: results after nine screening rounds. Scand J Gastroenterol 2004;39(9):846–51.

13. Lindholm E, Brevinge H, Haglind E. Survival benefit in a randomized clinical trial of faecal occult blood screening for colorectal cancer. Br J Surg 2008;95(8): 1029–36.

14. Scholefield JH, Moss SM, Mangham CM, et al. Nottingham trial of faecal occult blood testing for colorectal cancer: a 20-year follow-up. Gut 2012;61(7):1036–40.

15. Shaukat A, Mongin SJ, Geisser MS, et al. Long-term mortality after screening for colorectal cancer. N Engl J Med 2013;369(12):1106–14.

16. Mandel JS, Church TR, Bond JH, et al. The effect of fecal occult-blood screening on the incidence of colorectal cancer. N Engl J Med 2000;343(22):1603–7.

17. Allison JE, Tekawa IS, Ransom LJ, et al. A comparison of fecal occult-blood tests for colorectal-cancer screening. N Engl J Med 1996;334(3):155–9.

18. Levi Z, Birkenfeld S, Vilkin A, et al. A higher detection rate for colorectal cancer and advanced adenomatous polyp for screening with immunochemical fecal occult blood test than guaiac fecal occult blood test, despite lower compliance rate. A prospective, controlled, feasibility study. Int J Cancer 2011;128(10): 2415–24.

19. Ransohoff DF, Lang CA. Screening for colorectal cancer with the fecal occult blood test: a background paper. American College of Physicians. Ann Intern Med 1997;126(10):811–22.

20. Vart G, Banzi R, Minozzi S. Comparing participation rates between immunochemical and guaiac faecal occult blood tests: a systematic review and meta-analysis. Prev Med 2012;55(2):87–92.

21. Lee JK, Liles EG, Bent S, et al. Accuracy of fecal immunochemical tests for colorectal cancer: systematic review and meta-analysis. Ann Intern Med 2014; 160(3):171.

22. Robertson DJ, Lee JK, Boland CR, et al. Recommendations on fecal immuno-chemical testing to screen for colorectal neoplasia: a consensus statement by the US multi-society task force on colorectal cancer. Gastroenterology 2017; 152(5):1217–37.e3.

23. Imperiale TF, Ransohoff DF, Itzkowitz SH, et al. Multitarget stool DNA testing for colorectal-cancer screening. N Engl J Med 2014;370(14):1287–97.

24. Ladabaum U, Mannalithara A. Comparative effectiveness and cost effectiveness of a multitarget stool DNA test to screen for colorectal neoplasia. Gastroenterology 2016;151(3):427–39.e6.

25. Lin JS, Piper MA, Perdue LA, et al. Screening for colorectal cancer: a systematic review for the U.S. preventive services task force. Evidence Synthesis No. 135. Rockville (MD): Agency for Healthcare Research and Quality; 2015.

26. IJspeert JEG, Tutein Nolthenius CJ, Kuipers EJ, et al. CT-colonography vs. colonoscopy for detection of high-risk sessile serrated polyps. Am J Gastroenterol 2016;111(4):516–22.

27. Rex DK, Adler SN, Aisenberg J, et al. Accuracy of capsule colonoscopy in detecting colorectal polyps in a screening population. Gastroenterology 2015; 148(5):948–57.e2.

28. Church TR, Wandell M, Lofton-Day C, et al. Prospective evaluation of methylated SEPT9 in plasma for detection of asymptomatic colorectal cancer. Gut 2014; 63(2):317–25.

29. Potter NT, Hurban P, White MN, et al. Validation of a real-time PCR-based qualitative assay for the detection of methylated SEPT9 DNA in human plasma. Clin Chem 2014;60(9):1183–91.

30. Baxter NN, Warren JL, Barrett MJ, et al. Association between colonoscopy and colorectal cancer mortality in a US cohort according to site of cancer and colonoscopist specialty. J Clin Oncol 2012;30(21):2664–9.

31. Kahi CJ, Pohl H, Myers LJ, et al. Colonoscopy and colorectal cancer mortality in the veterans affairs health care system: a case-control study. Ann Intern Med 2018;168(7):481–8.

32. Nishihara R, Wu K, Lochhead P, et al. Long-term colorectal-cancer incidence and mortality after lower endoscopy. N Engl J Med 2013;369(12):1095–105.

33. Corley DA, Jensen CD, Marks AR, et al. Adenoma detection rate and risk of colorectal cancer and death. N Engl J Med 2014;370(14):1298–306.

34. Rex DK, Schoenfeld PS, Cohen J, et al. Quality indicators for colonoscopy. Am J Gastroenterol 2015;110(1):72–90.

35. Schoen RE, Pinsky PF, Weissfeld JL, et al. Colorectal-cancer incidence and mortality with screening flexible sigmoidoscopy. N Engl J Med 2012;366(25): 2345–57.

36. Segnan N, Armaroli P, Bonelli L, et al. Once-only sigmoidoscopy in colorectal cancer screening: follow-up findings of the Italian Randomized Controlled Trial–SCORE. J Natl Cancer Inst 2011;103(17):1310–22.

37. Atkin W, Wooldrage K, Parkin DM, et al. Long term effects of once-only flexible sigmoidoscopy screening after 17 years of follow-up: the UK Flexible Sigmoidoscopy Screening randomised controlled trial. Lancet 2017;389(10076):1299–311.

38. Holme Ø, Løberg M, Kalager M, et al. Long-term effectiveness of sigmoidoscopy screening on colorectal cancer incidence and mortality in women and men: a randomized trial. Ann Intern Med 2018;168(11):775–82.

39. US Preventive Services Task Force, Bibbins-Domingo K, Grossman DC, et al. Screening for colorectal cancer: US Preventive Services Task Force recommendation statement. JAMA 2016;315(23):2564–75.

40. Rex DK, Boland CR, Dominitz JA, et al. Colorectal cancer screening: recommendations for physicians and patients from the U.S. multi-society task force on colorectal cancer. Gastroenterology 2017;153(1):307–23.

41. Bacchus CM, Dunfield L, Gorber SC, et al. Recommendations on screening for colorectal cancer in primary care. CMAJ 2016;188(5):340–8.

42. Fitzpatrick-Lewis D, Usman A, Warren R, et al. Screening for colorectal cancer. Ottawa (Canada): Canadian Task Force on Preventive Health Care; 2015. Available at: https://canadiantaskforce.ca/wp-content/uploads/2016/03/crc-screeningfinal031216.pdf. Accessed May 1, 2018.

43. National Center for Health Statistics. National Health Interview Survey, 2015. Public-use data file and documentation. Available at: http://www.cdc.gov/nchs/nhis/quest_data_related_1997_forward.htm. Accessed May 1, 2018.

44. Liang PS, Wheat CL, Abhat A, et al. Adherence to competing strategies for colorectal cancer screening over 3 years. Am J Gastroenterol 2016;111(1):105–14.
45. Lansdorp-Vogelaar I, Knudsen AB, Brenner H. Cost-effectiveness of colorectal cancer screening. Epidemiol Rev 2011;33:88–100.
46. Knudsen AB, Zauber AG, Rutter CM, et al. Estimation of benefits, burden, and harms of colorectal cancer screening strategies: modeling study for the US preventive services task force. JAMA 2016;315(23):2595–609.
47. Reumkens A, Rondagh EJA, Bakker CM, et al. Post-colonoscopy complications: a systematic review, time trends, and meta-analysis of population-based studies. Am J Gastroenterol 2016;111(8):1092–101.
48. Goodwin JS, Singh A, Reddy N, et al. Overuse of screening colonoscopy in the Medicare population. Arch Intern Med 2011;171(15):1335–43.
49. Lieberman DA, Williams JL, Holub JL, et al. Colonoscopy utilization and outcomes 2000 to 2011. Gastrointest Endosc 2014;80(1):133–43.
50. Lieberman DA, Rex DK, Winawer SJ, et al. Guidelines for colonoscopy surveillance after screening and polypectomy: a consensus update by the US Multi-Society Task Force on Colorectal Cancer. Gastroenterology 2012;143(3):844–57.
51. Johnson MR, Grubber J, Grambow SC, et al. Physician non-adherence to colonoscopy interval guidelines in the veterans affairs healthcare system. Gastroenterology 2015;149(4):938–51.
52. Click B, Pinsky PF, Hickey T, et al. Association of colonoscopy adenoma findings with long-term colorectal cancer incidence. JAMA 2018;319(19):2021.
53. Jover R, Bretthauer M, Dekker E, et al. Rationale and design of the European Polyp Surveillance (EPoS) trials. Endoscopy 2016;48(6):571–8.
54. Corley DA, Jensen CD, Quinn VP, et al. Association between time to colonoscopy after a positive fecal test result and risk of colorectal cancer and cancer stage at diagnosis. JAMA 2017;317(16):1631–41.
55. Inadomi JM, Vijan S, Janz NK, et al. Adherence to colorectal cancer screening: a randomized clinical trial of competing strategies. Arch Intern Med 2012;172(7):575–82.
56. Holme Ø, Løberg M, Kalager M, et al. Effect of flexible sigmoidoscopy screening on colorectal cancer incidence and mortality: a randomized clinical trial. JAMA 2014;312(6):606–15.

Colonoscopy, Polypectomy, and the Risk of Bleeding

Linda Anne Feagins, MD

KEYWORDS

- Polypectomy • Gastrointestinal hemorrhage • Colonoscopy • Risks
- Antiplatelet agents • Anticoagulants

KEY POINTS

- There is no need to withdraw cardioprotective aspirin for polypectomy.
- Avoid withdrawing either aspirin or thienopyridines within 30 days of cardiac stenting and consider postponing elective colonoscopy up to 12 months if feasible after placement of drug-eluting stents.
- If feasible, consider postponing elective colonoscopy until short-term anticoagulant treatment is completed.
- Do not withdraw antiplatelets or anticoagulants for low-risk bleeding procedures (ie, diagnostic colonoscopy with no polypectomy).
- For colonoscopy with polypectomy, withdraw thienopyridines for 5–7 days and continue aspirin; withdraw warfarin for 5 days; and withdraw direct-acting oral anticoagulants for 1–2 days if kidney function is normal, or longer if kidney function is abnormal.

INTRODUCTION

Colorectal cancer will occur in 1 in 22 men (4.5%) and 1 in 24 women (4.2%) over a lifetime. Moreover, colorectal cancer is the third leading cause of cancer deaths in the United States.[1] The 5-year survival after the diagnosis with colorectal cancer is better for patients diagnosed with cancer in an early stage as opposed to those detected in a more advanced or metastatic stage. Fortunately, colorectal cancer usually arises slowly over time. Screening programs can detect the cancer early or even prevent it through the removal of polyps via colonoscopy.

RISKS OF COLONOSCOPY

Although colonoscopy is generally considered a safe procedure, it is not without risks. Risks of colonoscopy include perforation, hemorrhage, complications of sedation,

Dr. Feagins current research is funded by a VA CSR&D MERIT Award grant number 5I01CX00815.
Division of Gastroenterology and Hepatology, University of Texas Southwestern Medical Center, VA North Texas Healthcare System, Dallas VA Medical Center, 4500 South Lancaster Road (111B1), Dallas, TX 75216, USA
E-mail address: Linda.Feagins@UTSouthwestern.edu

Med Clin N Am 103 (2019) 125–135
https://doi.org/10.1016/j.mcna.2018.08.003
0025-7125/19/Published by Elsevier Inc.

postpolypectomy coagulation syndrome, and (rarely) splenic rupture (**Table 1**). Indeed, colonoscopic complications (particularly perforation or hemorrhage) occur most commonly in patients who undergo polypectomy.[2] Hemorrhage after removal of a polyp, termed postpolypectomy bleeding (PPB), can occur in 1 of 2 forms: immediate PPB (occurring during the procedure) and delayed PPB (occurring at some time after completion of the procedure, usually within 1–2 weeks).[3] Immediate PPB is thought to be caused by inadequate cauterization of the polyp vessels during polypectomy and occurs in 1% to 2% of polypectomies.[4] Immediate bleeding is readily controlled during the colonoscopy with various hemostatic techniques, including the placement of hemoclips.[5,6] Delayed PPB is thought to be due to the sloughing of the eschar of a cautery-induced ulcer, with exposure and penetration of an underlying vessel. Delayed PPB is considered clinically important if it results in hospitalization or blood transfusion, or if repeat colonoscopy or surgery is performed to treat the bleeding site.[2]

RISK FACTORS FOR POSTPOLYPECTOMY BLEEDING

Polyp factors, patient factors, and even physician factors have been associated with an increased risk of immediate and/or delayed PPB.[7–10] Polyp-related factors include polyp size, polyp morphology, and polyp location in the colon. One of the major polyp-related risk factors for PPB is polyp size. In a study investigating pedunculated polyps, the PPB rate (immediate or delayed) for 98 polyps that were 1 to 1.9 cm was 3.1%, whereas PPB occurred in 15.1% of 66 polyps 2 cm or greater.[11] In a retrospective study of 9336 colonic polypectomies, a multivariate analysis of risk factors for immediate PPB found polyp size greater than 1 cm to be a significant risk factor for bleeding, with an odds ratio (OR) of 2.4.[10] Moreover, another study with a case-control design evaluating delayed PPB found that for every 1 mm increase in polyp diameter, the risk of hemorrhage increased by 9%.[9] Increased risk for PPB has also been associated with the morphology of the polyp, including pedunculated polyps or laterally spreading tumors and polyps located on the right side of the colon.[9]

Patient-related factors that increase the risk of PPB include age over 65 years, history of cardiovascular disease, and the use of antiplatelet agents (thienopyridines) and anticoagulants (warfarin). A retrospective cohort study specifically focused on the use of periprocedural anticoagulation found that delayed PPB occurred in 2.6% of subjects with interrupted warfarin for polypectomy as compared with 0.2% of subjects not taking any anticoagulation (OR = 11.6, P = .005).[8] A meta-analysis found that polypectomy on uninterrupted clopidogrel increased the risk of delayed PPB (relative risk 4.66, CI 2.37–9.17, P<.00001).[12] Although thienopyridines and warfarin have been shown to increase the risk of PPB, it is important to remember that the risk of PPB

Table 1 Common complications associated with screening colonoscopy	
Complication	Risk (%)
Perforation	<0.1
Hemorrhage	0.1–0.6
Cardiopulmonary complications	0.9
Postpolypectomy electrocoagulation syndrome	0.1–0.003

has not been shown to increase with the use of aspirin or nonsteroidal antiinflammatory drugs (NSAIDs) alone.[13]

Finally, physician-related factors for PPB include the techniques chosen for the removal of polyps. The use of snare with electrocautery (hot snare) as opposed to snare with no cautery (cold snare) is thought to carry a higher risk for delayed PPB. Although this has not been well-studied for the removal of large polyps, several case series have reported very low rates of delayed bleeding after removal with cold snare.[14,15] Another technique, prophylactic hemoclipping, has gained popularity in recent years with the thought that the routine placement of hemoclips after polypectomy, especially for large polyps, may reduce the risk of delayed bleeding.[16] However, aside from 1 retrospective study that showed promise, this practice has yet to be confirmed to be beneficial in randomized trials.[17–19] A large randomized multisite trial of hemoclipping after removing large polyps is currently underway at the author's organization, the Veterans Affairs North Texas Healthcare System, with results expected in the next 1 to 2 years.

OUTCOMES OF PATIENTS WITH POSTPOLYPECTOMY BLEEDING

Fortunately, for patients who do experience PPB, this complication is not typically associated with any major long-term sequelae. In a study of 1657 subjects undergoing polypectomy, there were 5 with delayed PPB, all of whom received blood transfusion. Four of the 5 were treated successfully endoscopically, and PPB was controlled in the fifth with angiography after endoscopic treatment had failed. None of these subjects required surgery and none died of PPB.[20] In the author's study, thienopyridines were not withdrawn before polypectomy for 219 subjects. Of these, 5 experienced delayed PPB, all of whom were treated successfully with either expectant management or endoscopic treatment, with no need for angiography or surgery, and no deaths.[7]

CONSIDERATIONS WHEN REFERRING PATIENTS FOR COLONOSCOPY

When referring patients for colonoscopy, it is very important to carefully evaluate their regimen of antiplatelets or anticoagulants and the timing of the colonoscopy. The use of antiplatelets and anticoagulants is increasing given the high rates of coronary artery disease and cerebrovascular disease in the United States. The American Heart Association estimates that 83.6 million American adults have some form of cardiovascular disease, including approximately 15.4 million with coronary artery disease and 6.8 million with strokes.[21] When considering a colonoscopy, the risks of withdrawing these drugs, and thus precipitating thrombotic events, must be carefully weighed against the risks of continuing these agents during endoscopic procedures that can be complicated by bleeding, particularly procedures with high bleeding risk interventions such as polypectomy. Moreover, when treatment with agents that increase the risk of bleeding is short-term, elective procedures should be delayed until therapy is completed. It must also be kept in mind that, although polypectomy does carry a risk for hemorrhage, many of the patients who are undergoing colonoscopy for colon cancer screening or surveillance will not require a polypectomy during their colonoscopy; however, this is not known until the procedure is completed. When considering endoscopy for patients taking anticoagulants, several important issues should be weighed (**Box 1**).

MANAGING ASPIRIN IN THE PERIPROCEDURAL PERIOD

Aspirin irreversibly acetylates and inactivates the platelet cyclooxygenase, thereby inactivating platelets for the duration of their lifespan, 7 to 10 days. Nevertheless,

> **Box 1**
> **Questions to consider when evaluating a patient on anticoagulants or antiplatelet agents for colonoscopy**
>
> How urgent is the procedure?
>
> Does the colonoscopy really need to be performed immediately, or could the patient safely wait several months until the anticoagulants might be withdrawn and/or the risk for thrombotic events may be less?
>
> What is the risk of bleeding (related to the drug and to the planned procedure)?
>
> Is the procedure likely to be diagnostic only or likely to include an intervention that has a high risk of bleeding?
>
> What is the risk of drug interruption (ie, thromboembolic event)?
>
> Is the risk of a thromboembolic event greater than that of a bleeding complication from the endoscopic procedure?
>
> If the drug is withdrawn temporarily, what is the optimal timing of withdrawing and readministering the drug, and does the drug need to be reloaded?
>
> Should the drug be withdrawn for all patients undergoing endoscopy when there is potential for a high-risk intervention, or should the agent be continued with a plan to perform another endoscopy off drug only if a lesion requiring a high-risk intervention is found?

based on several retrospective studies,[13,20,22] guidelines agree that aspirin can be safely continued during colonoscopy with polypectomy without concern for a significant increase in bleeding.[23–25] Moreover, the cardiovascular risks associated with withdrawing aspirin can be high, especially in patients with a history of coronary artery disease. One group polled 1236 subjects who were hospitalized for acute coronary syndromes regarding recent aspirin use.[26] They found that 51 cases of acute coronary syndrome occurred within 1 month of withdrawing aspirin (4.1% of all cases and 13% of recurrences), with 20% associated with late stent thrombosis (average 15 months after stent placement). Another study found that recent cessation of antiplatelet agents (mostly for elective surgery) in subjects with acute coronary syndromes was associated with higher 30-day rates of death or myocardial infarction than in subjects who had only a remote history of aspirin use.[27]

MANAGING THIENOPYRIDINES IN THE PERIPROCEDURAL PERIOD

The thienopyridines inhibit platelet function by blocking adenosine diphosphate, which interferes with the platelets' ability to aggregate. In patients with coronary artery disease, especially in the setting of coronary stents, thienopyridines are most frequently given in combination with aspirin, which is termed dual antiplatelet therapy (DAPT). For patients on continued thienopyridines during polypectomy, prospective data found the rate of PPB to be 2.4% and interestingly, all patients with the complication of bleeding where on both a thienopyridine and concomitant aspirin.[7] Although PPB is a complication best avoided, it is important to note that this complication has low associated mortality, is usually managed without surgery, and has no long-term consequences. Although not trivial, this must be compared with the outcomes of thromboembolic events related to withdrawing antiplatelet agents, including stent thrombosis. One study of 2229 subjects with drug-eluting coronary stents found that, for subjects who had the complication of stent thrombosis, the mortality rate was 45%.[28] Although the highest risk period for stent thrombosis is within the first 30 days after stent placement, it is now well-accepted that there remains a substantial prolonged risk for delayed stent thrombosis, particularly in patients with drug-eluting stents (DESs).[29,30] For bare-metal stents, the highest risk period is within the first 30 days after stent placement. However, for DESs, which undergo delayed endothelialization, high risk for stent thrombosis continues for at least 6 months, with a lower but considerable risk for late thrombosis extending 12 to 24 months.[31] To date, there have not been any studies that specifically have evaluated the risk of cardiovascular events associated with the interruption of thienopyridine therapy for endoscopic procedures. However, a systematic review of 161 subjects with late stent thrombosis found that the practice of continuing aspirin therapy when withdrawing clopidogrel increased the time to stent thrombosis from 7 days to 122 days. However, 6% of the subjects who developed a stent thrombosis while taking aspirin did so within 10 days of withdrawing clopidogrel.[29] Therefore, although the practice of continuing aspirin when clopidogrel is withdrawn substantially reduces the risk of stent thrombosis, the practice is not risk-free.

The 2016 American Society for Gastrointestinal Endoscopy (ASGE) guidelines for the periprocedural management of thienopyridines recommend, in general, cessation of thienopyridines while continuing aspirin when planned procedures include a high risk for bleeding, such as polypectomy.[32] However, for high-risk thromboembolic conditions, consideration should be given to postponing the procedure until the risk of discontinuing thienopyridines is lower (eg, waiting up to 12 months after placement of a drug-eluting coronary stent). Moreover, the urgency of the procedure needs to be weighed into the timing of the procedure. For example, postponing referral of a patient for a screening or surveillance procedure until 12 months of DAPT (for a patient with a DES) is ideal, whereas waiting only 6 months of therapy after a DES placement may be preferred for an asymptomatic patient with iron deficiency anemia. Consideration should also be given to performing the procedure on uninterrupted thienopyridines after a careful weighing of risks and benefits if there is a high urgency for the procedure. Moreover, for endoscopic procedures that are considered low risk for bleeding (eg, diagnostic colonoscopy to evaluate iron deficiency anemia with no plan for polypectomy), the ASGE recommendation is to continue the agents during the procedure. If postponement is deemed inadvisable or unlikely to affect the risk of thromboembolism and the planned procedure is high-risk for bleeding, then the thienopyridine should be discontinued 5 to 7 days before the procedure. Finally, of interest, studies have explored using other short-acting anticoagulants for bridging while off thienopyridines, including heparin, glycoprotein IIb/IIIa inhibitors, and short-acting platelet P2Y12 inhibitors; however, none have had favorable outcomes to date.

MANAGING WARFARIN IN THE PERIPROCEDURAL PERIOD

Warfarin is a commonly used anticoagulant agent that works by inhibiting vitamin K–dependent coagulation factor synthesis. This drug is used for treatment of a variety of disorders, including deep vein thrombosis (DVT); pulmonary embolism; ischemic stroke; and prophylaxis of arterial thromboembolism from atrial fibrillation, flutter, and cardiac valvular disorders. It is important to remember that, although the goal with interrupting anticoagulants periprocedurally is to reduce the risk of bleeding, patients who are on warfarin therapy are still at increased risk for bleeding postprocedure despite withdrawing the drug periprocedurally. A retrospective study compared delayed PPB in subjects who interrupted their warfarin to subjects who were not on warfarin and found significantly higher rates of bleeding in those who used warfarin despite it being withdrawn for the procedures (OR = 11.6, 2.6% vs 0.2%, CI 2.3–57.3, P = .005).[8] A few studies have even evaluated performing polypectomy for subjects on therapeutic warfarin, although this has not been the standard for most practices. One group reviewed their experience of removing small (<10 mm) polyps while the patients were on therapeutic warfarin and reported a delayed PPB rate of 0.8%.[33] Further, subjects who took heparin as a bridge while their warfarin was interrupted were at higher risk for bleeding compared with subjects who were on warfarin that was not bridged (20% vs 1.4%, bridged vs not bridged, respectively).[34] Currently, for patients with nonvalvular atrial fibrillation, scores such as the CHADS$_2$ are used to determine the risk for stroke and to help determine if bridging therapy is needed periprocedurally. The risks of thromboembolic events during warfarin cessation for colonoscopy have not been extensively studied. One study, however, reviewed subjects with atrial fibrillation who were on warfarin and were undergoing endoscopy (esophagogastroduodenoscopy, colonoscopy, or bronchoscopy). They found that in 987 subjects undergoing 1137 procedures, 12 subjects experienced strokes within 30 days (1.06%/procedure) as compared with no strokes in 438 subjects who did not have their warfarin adjusted. Moreover, the stroke risk was greatest for the subjects undergoing more complex procedures or with more comorbid illness.[35]

Similar to the ASGE recommendations for antiplatelet agents, the decision whether to withdraw or continue the warfarin during endoscopy is based on an assessment of bleeding risk from the planned procedure, the thromboembolic risk if the drug is withdrawn, and the urgency of the procedure. If the procedure is low risk for bleeding (eg, a diagnostic colonoscopy with no plan for polypectomy), the warfarin may be continued during the procedure. Specifically, mucosal biopsy is safe to perform during endoscopy for patients on warfarin whose international normalized ratio (INR) is in the therapeutic range.[36] However, current guidelines recommend that, for high risk procedures such as polypectomy, warfarin should be discontinued for 5 days before the procedure. When the decision is made to discontinue the warfarin, the risk for thromboembolic disease must be weighed in the decision whether or not to bridge the warfarin with a short-acting anticoagulant such as unfractionated heparin or low-molecular-weight heparin. For high thromboembolic risk conditions, consideration should be given to postponing the procedure, particularly if the treatment duration of the anticoagulant may soon be reached (eg, waiting for completion of 6 months of warfarin for a provoked DVT). If postponement is deemed inadvisable or unlikely to affect the risk of thromboembolism, then the warfarin should be discontinued and bridging begun. For patients who were on warfarin that was bridged, heparin was administered when the INR is 2 or less. The heparin should then be discontinued 4 to 6 hours before the procedure for unfractionated heparin, or withdrawn the day before the procedure (ie, last dose 24 hours before the procedure) for low-molecular-weight heparin.

MANAGING DIRECT-ACTING ORAL ANTICOAGULANTS IN THE PERIPROCEDURAL PERIOD

The direct-acting oral anticoagulants (DOACs) include the direct thrombin inhibitor, dabigatran; and the factor Xa inhibitors, rivaroxaban, apixaban, edoxaban, and betrixaban. Additionally, there are subcutaneous and intravenous direct thrombin inhibitors and factor Xa inhibitors (**Table 2**); however, this article focuses on the oral agents because they are the drugs most likely to be encountered in the setting of elective colonoscopy. The major advantages of the DOACs compared with warfarin are the lack of requirement for monitoring with blood tests, fewer interactions with diet and other medications, and quicker onset and washout of action (with normal kidney function). On the other hand, these agents are more expensive than warfarin and, with the exception of dabigatran, there is no available means to reverse their anticoagulant

Table 2
Currently approved direct thrombin inhibitors and factor Xa inhibitors

Drug	Mechanism	Approved Indications
Dabigatran (oral)	Direct thrombin inhibitor	Prophylaxis of thromboembolic events in nonvalvular atrial fibrillation
Desirudin (subcutaneous)	Direct thrombin inhibitor	DVT or pulmonary embolism (PE) prophylaxis in patients undergoing elective hip replacement
Argatroban (intravenous)	Direct thrombin inhibitor	Adjunct anticoagulants for percutaneous coronary interventions
Bivalirudin (intravenous)	Direct thrombin inhibitor	Adjunct anticoagulants for percutaneous coronary interventions
Rivaroxaban (oral)	Factor Xa inhibitor	Stroke prophylaxis in patients with nonvalvular atrial fibrillation, the prevention of DVT and PE after hip and knee replacement surgery, and for acute treatment of DVT and PE
Apixaban (oral)	Factor Xa inhibitor	Stroke prophylaxis in patients with nonvalvular atrial fibrillation
Edoxaban (oral)	Factor Xa inhibitor	Stroke prophylaxis in patients with nonvalvular atrial fibrillation
Betrixaban (oral)	Factor Xa inhibitor	VTE prophylaxis in acutely hospitalized patients
Fondaparinux (subcutaneous)	Factor Xa inhibitor	DVT and PE prophylaxis in patients undergoing hip, knee or abdominal surgery, and for treatment of acute DVT and PE when administered with warfarin

effects in the event of bleeding. Similar to warfarin, the DOACs increase the risk of bleeding from all causes. Unrelated to polypectomy, the rate of gastrointestinal (GI) bleeding was higher for subjects treated with dabigatran[37] (3% vs 2%), rivaroxaban[38] (3.2% vs 2.2%), or edoxaban[39] (1.5% vs 1.2%) as compared with subjects taking warfarin. On the other hand, the rates of GI bleeding were similar if not lower for subjects treated with apixaban[40] as compared with warfarin (1.2% vs 1.3%). The reason for the increased risk of GI bleeding with many of the DOACs is not clear but may be related to the activation of dabigatran in the distal bowel. It has been proposed that this active drug in the distal bowel may promote GI bleeding more than warfarin, which is not activated in the bowel.[41] There also are reports of dabigatran use being associated with esophagitis and gastric ulceration, and it has been proposed that the drug may cause direct injury to GI mucosae.[42,43] No studies have specifically explored bleeding rates with high-risk endoscopic procedures such as polypectomy; however, a small Japanese study did find that endoscopic mucosal biopsy seems to be safe for patients taking dabigatran.[36] Moreover, a post hoc analysis of the Randomized Evaluation of Long-Term Anticoagulation Therapy (RE-LY) study (the randomized controlled trial that gained dabigatran its approval from the US Food and Drug Administration) found no significant differences in rates of periprocedural bleeding between subjects taking warfarin and subjects taking dabigatran; however, only 8.6% of the procedures were colonoscopies.[44]

The most recent ASGE guidelines (2016) include recommendations on the management of the DOACs in the periprocedural period. As with other antiplatelet agents and anticoagulants, for procedures with low bleeding risk, the DOACs can likely be continued safely throughout the periprocedural period. For procedures with high bleeding risk, such as polypectomy, the DOACs should be withdrawn before the procedure. Given the quick onset and washout (with normal renal function) of these agents, there is no need for periprocedural bridging. The guidelines recommend holding these agents for 2 to 3 half-lives before the procedure (1–2 days). For patients with mild to moderate kidney disease (creatinine clearance <50 mL/min), the drug should be withdrawn 3 to 5 days before the procedure. Generally, postprocedure, the agent can be readministered immediately or within several days, depending on the bleeding risk for the intervention that was performed.

WHEN TO READMINISTER DRUGS AFTER THE PROCEDURE

After making the decision to discontinue an antiplatelet or anticoagulant in preparation for an endoscopic procedure, the next important decision is when to readminister the drug after the procedure. Unfortunately, the guidelines provide no clear consensus because there are very few studies on which to base the recommendations. For thienopyridines, the ACC/ACG (the joint guidelines from the American College of Cardiology and American College of Gastroenterology) recommend readministering "as soon as possible," the ASGE recommends timing based on weighing the risks of thromboembolic disease with holding the medication and risks of bleeding based on the procedure performed with readministering immediately, and the British Society of Gastroenterology recommends readministering the day after the procedure. All of these recommendations are based on opinion because there are no definitive data to guide these decisions. When readministering a thienopyridine, another contentious issue is whether reloading of the drug (to obtain quicker therapeutic levels) is necessary. When readministering clopidogrel in its usual oral dose (75 mg per day), it takes 5 to 10 days to reach maximal platelet inhibition, compared with 12 to 15 hours if the patient is given a 300 to 600 mg loading dose. The JACC/ACG guideline recommends that the decision regarding the need for reloading should be tailored to the patient's thromboembolic risk. Studies of subjects who had percutaneous intervention for coronary artery disease did not reveal significant differences in adverse outcomes, including bleeding, between subjects who received loading doses of thienopyridines and those who received standard dosing.[45] No comparable data are available for endoscopic procedures.

For patients who were on warfarin that was not bridged, the ASGE guidelines recommend readministering warfarin within 24 hours. For patients who were on warfarin that was bridged, warfarin should be readministered on the evening of the procedure, whereas heparin should be resumed as soon as possible after the procedure and withdrawn once the INR has become therapeutic. However, adjustment to these guidelines may be necessary on a case by case basis in the setting of high-risk bleeding procedures, such as large polypectomies, because a case-control study found that even resuming warfarin within 7 days of polypectomy was a risk factor for PPB.[9]

For patients on DOACs, the ASGE recommends these agents also should be readministered as soon as possible. In cases in which they cannot be readministered within 24 hours due to concern for high risk of bleeding, consideration should be given to administering a heparin bridge for those at high thromboembolic risk.

SUMMARY

Colonoscopy with polypectomy is the means by which the incidence of colon cancer may be reduced; however, polypectomy is not without risk. Physicians must carefully weigh the risks and benefits of colonoscopy, particularly when patients are prescribed antiplatelet agents and anticoagulants. Aspirin and NSAIDs can be continued safely during colonoscopy with polypectomy. The risk of delayed PPB is increased if thieno-pyridines are continued and is increased even if warfarin therapy is interrupted. For the thienopyridines, warfarin and the new novel oral anticoagulants, the decision to inter-rupt or continue these agents for endoscopy involves considerable exercise of clinical judgment.

REFERENCES

1. American Cancer Society. Colorectal cancer facts & figures 2017-2019. Atlanta (GA): American Cancer Society; 2017.
2. ASGE Standards of Practice Committee, Fisher DA, Maple JT, Ben-Menachem T, et al. Complications of colonoscopy. Gastrointest Endosc 2011;74:745–52.
3. Gibbs DH, Opelka FG, Beck DE, et al. Postpolypectomy colonic hemorrhage. Dis Colon Rectum 1996;39:806–10.
4. Waye JD, Lewis BS, Yessayan S. Colonoscopy: a prospective report of complica-tions. J Clin Gastroenterol 1992;15:347–51.
5. Parra-Blanco A, Kaminaga N, Kojima T, et al. Hemoclipping for postpolypectomy and postbiopsy colonic bleeding. Gastrointest Endosc 2000;51:37–41.
6. Tolliver KA, Rex DK. Colonoscopic polypectomy. Gastroenterol Clin North Am 2008;37:229–51, ix.
7. Feagins LA, Iqbal R, Harford WV, et al. Low rate of postpolypectomy bleeding among patients who continue thienopyridine therapy during colonoscopy. Clin Gastroenterol Hepatol 2013;11:1325–32.
8. Witt DM, Delate T, McCool KH, et al. Incidence and predictors of bleeding or thrombosis after polypectomy in patients receiving and not receiving anticoagu-lation therapy. J Thromb Haemost 2009;7:1982–9.
9. Sawhney MS, Salfiti N, Nelson DB, et al. Risk factors for severe delayed postpo-lypectomy bleeding. Endoscopy 2008;40:115–9.
10. Kim HS, Kim TI, Kim WH, et al. Risk factors for immediate postpolypectomy bleeding of the colon: a multicenter study. Am J Gastroenterol 2006;101:1333–41.
11. Di Giorgio P, De Luca L, Calcagno G, et al. Detachable snare versus epinephrine injection in the prevention of postpolypectomy bleeding: a randomized and controlled study. Endoscopy 2004;36:860–3.
12. Gandhi S, Narula N, Mosleh W, et al. Meta-analysis: colonoscopic post-polypectomy bleeding in patients on continued clopidogrel therapy. Aliment Pharmacol Ther 2013;37:947–52.
13. Yousfi M, Gostout CJ, Baron TH, et al. Postpolypectomy lower gastrointestinal bleeding: potential role of aspirin. Am J Gastroenterol 2004;99:1785–9.
14. Muniraj T, Sahakian A, Ciarleglio MM, et al. Cold snare polypectomy for large sessile colonic polyps: a single-center experience. Gastroenterol Res Pract 2015;2015:175959.
15. Choksi N, Elmunzer BJ, Stidham RW, et al. Cold snare piecemeal resection of colonic and duodenal polyps >/=1 cm. Endosc Int Open 2015;3:E508–13.
16. Feagins LA, Spechler SJ. Use of hemoclips and other measures to prevent bleeding during colonoscopy by gastroenterologists in Veterans Affairs hospitals. Am J Gastroenterol 2014;109:288–90.
17. Shioji K, Suzuki Y, Kobayashi M, et al. Prophylactic clip application does not decrease delayed bleeding after colonoscopic polypectomy. Gastrointest En-dosc 2003;57:691–4.

18. Liaquat H, Rohn E, Rex DK. Prophylactic clip closure reduced the risk of delayed postpolypectomy hemorrhage: experience in 277 clipped large sessile or flat colorectal lesions and 247 control lesions. Gastrointest Endosc 2013;77:401–7.

19. Quintanilla E, Castro JL, Rábago LR, et al. Is the use of prophylactic hemoclips in the endoscopic resection of large pedunculated polyps useful? A prospective and randomized study. J Interv Gastroenterol 2012;2:183–8.

20. Hui AJ, Wong RM, Ching JY, et al. Risk of colonoscopic polypectomy bleeding with anticoagulants and antiplatelet agents: analysis of 1657 cases. Gastrointest Endosc 2004;59:44–8.

21. Go AS, Mozaffarian D, Roger VL, et al. Heart disease and stroke statistics–2014 update: a report from the American Heart Association. Circulation 2014;129: e28–292.

22. Shiffman ML, Farrel MT, Yee YS. Risk of bleeding after endoscopic biopsy or polypectomy in patients taking aspirin or other NSAIDS. Gastrointest Endosc 1994; 40:458–62.

23. Veitch AM, Baglin TP, Gershlick AH, et al. Guidelines for the management of anticoagulant and antiplatelet therapy in patients undergoing endoscopic procedures. Gut 2008;57:1322–9.

24. Becker RC, Scheiman J, Dauerman HL, et al. Management of platelet-directed pharmacotherapy in patients with atherosclerotic coronary artery disease undergoing elective endoscopic gastrointestinal procedures. Am J Gastroenterol 2009; 104:2903–17.

25. ASGE Standards of Practice Committee, Anderson MA, Ben-Menachem T, Gan SI, et al. Management of antithrombotic agents for endoscopic procedures. Gastrointest Endosc 2009;70:1060–70.

26. Ferrari E, Benhamou M, Cerboni P, et al. Coronary syndromes following aspirin withdrawal: a special risk for late stent thrombosis. J Am Coll Cardiol 2005;45: 456–9.

27. Collet JP, Montalescot G, Blanchet B, et al. Impact of prior use or recent withdrawal of oral antiplatelet agents on acute coronary syndromes. Circulation 2004;110:2361–7.

28. Iakovou I, Schmidt T, Bonizzoni E, et al. Incidence, predictors, and outcome of thrombosis after successful implantation of drug-eluting stents. JAMA 2005; 293:2126–30.

29. Eisenberg MJ, Richard PR, Libersan D, et al. Safety of short-term discontinuation of antiplatelet therapy in patients with drug-eluting stents. Circulation 2009;119: 1634–42.

30. van Werkum JW, Heestermans AA, de Korte FI, et al. Long-term clinical outcome after a first angiographically confirmed coronary stent thrombosis: an analysis of 431 cases. Circulation 2009;119:828–34.

31. Darvish-Kazem S, Gandhi M, Marcucci M, et al. Perioperative management of antiplatelet therapy in patients with a coronary stent who need noncardiac surgery: a systematic review of clinical practice guidelines. Chest 2013;144: 1848–56.

32. ASGE Standards of Practice Committee, Acosta RD, Abraham NS, Chandrasekhara V, et al. The management of antithrombotic agents for patients undergoing GI endoscopy. Gastrointest Endosc 2016;83:3–16.

33. Friedland S, Sedehi D, Soetikno R. Colonoscopic polypectomy in anticoagulated patients. World J Gastroenterol 2009;15:1973–6.

34. Inoue T, Nishida T, Maekawa A, et al. Clinical features of post-polypectomy bleeding associated with heparin bridge therapy. Dig Endosc 2014;26:243–9.

35. Blacker DJ, Wijdicks EF, McClelland RL. Stroke risk in anticoagulated patients with atrial fibrillation undergoing endoscopy. Neurology 2003;61:964–8.
36. Fujita M, Shiotani A, Murao T, et al. Safety of gastrointestinal endoscopic biopsy in patients taking antithrombotics. Dig Endosc 2015;27(1):25–9.
37. Connolly SJ, Ezekowitz MD, Yusuf S, et al. Dabigatran versus warfarin in patients with atrial fibrillation. N Engl J Med 2009;361:1139–51.
38. Patel MR, Mahaffey KW, Garg J, et al. Rivaroxaban versus warfarin in nonvalvular atrial fibrillation. N Engl J Med 2011;365:883–91.
39. Giugliano RP, Ruff CT, Braunwald E, et al. Edoxaban versus warfarin in patients with atrial fibrillation. N Engl J Med 2013;369:2093–104.
40. Granger CB, Alexander JH, McMurray JJ, et al. Apixaban versus warfarin in patients with atrial fibrillation. N Engl J Med 2011;365:981–92.
41. Feagins LA, Weideman RA. GI bleeding risk of DOACs versus Warfarin: is newer better? Dig Dis Sci 2018;63(7):1675–7.
42. Ootani A, Hayashi Y, Miyagi Y. Dabigatran-induced esophagitis. Clin Gastroenterol Hepatol 2014;12:e55–6.
43. Singh S, Savage L, Klein M, et al. Severe necrotic oesophageal and gastric ulceration associated with dabigatran. BMJ Case Rep 2013;2013 [pii:bcr2013009139].
44. Healey JS, Eikelboom J, Douketis J, et al. Periprocedural bleeding and thromboembolic events with dabigatran compared with warfarin: results from the Randomized Evaluation of Long-Term Anticoagulation Therapy (RE-LY) randomized trial. Circulation 2012;126:343–8.
45. Patti G, Colonna G, Pasceri V, et al. Randomized trial of high loading dose of clopidogrel for reduction of periprocedural myocardial infarction in patients undergoing coronary intervention: results from the ARMYDA-2 (Antiplatelet therapy for Reduction of MYocardial Damage during Angioplasty) study. Circulation 2005;111:2099–106.

Irritable Bowel Syndrome
What Treatments Really Work

Nuha Alammar, MBBS[a], Ellen Stein, MD[b],*

KEYWORDS

- Irritable bowel syndrome (IBS) • Rome criteria • Constipation • Diarrhea

KEY POINTS

- Rome IV classification divides IBS into subtypes based on the predominant stool pattern.
- Dietary interventions, such as FODMAP-reduced diets, can be successful short-term treatments for patients with IBS.
- Mind-body techniques such as hypnotherapy can improve symptom management in IBS.
- Targeted symptomatic relief for the patient's predominant symptoms provides relief. In addition to effective older medications that are inexpensive and reliable, there are also newer treatments for IBS-D such as eluxadoline, and IBS-C with linaclotide, lubiprostone, plecanatide, which also can provide durable relief.

INTRODUCTION

Irritable bowel syndrome (IBS) is a disorder of the gastrointestinal tract characterized by chronic abdominal pain and altered bowel habits in the absence of demonstrable organic disease.[1,2] Although only 10% of patients with IBS seek medical attention,[3] it is one of the most common diseases treated. In the United States, IBS accounts for 25% to 50% of all referrals to gastroenterologists[4]; however, 40% of individuals who meet diagnostic criteria for IBS do not receive a formal diagnosis.[5]

EPIDEMIOLOGY

It is estimated that IBS affects approximately 5% to 15% of Western populations.[6] Lovell and Ford[7] conducted a meta-analysis of the literature that demonstrated that IBS is seen predominantly in women, with onset in those younger than 50 years, with a global prevalence of 11.2%.

Disclosure Statement: No disclosures for either author.
a Department of Medicine, Division of Gastroenterology, King Khalid University Hospital, King Saud University, P.O. Box 2925, Riyadh 11461, Saudi Arabia; b Department of Medicine, Division of Gastroenterology, Johns Hopkins University, 4940 Eastern Avenue, 3rd Floor, Baltimore, MD 21224, USA
* Corresponding author.
E-mail address: estein6@jhmi.edu

Med Clin N Am 103 (2019) 137–152
https://doi.org/10.1016/j.mcna.2018.08.006
0025-7125/19/© 2018 Elsevier Inc. All rights reserved.

medical.theclinics.com

CLINICAL PRESENTATION

IBS can present with a wide range of gastrointestinal symptoms. Although abdominal pain is among the most common symptoms, patients with IBS may also experience bloating, a sensation of incomplete evacuation, urgency, diarrhea, straining, and constipation.[8] Abdominal pain in IBS is usually crampy in nature with variable location and intensity.[9] The pain is related to bowel movements, with relief of pain after bowel movements for some patients, and pain worsening while having a bowel movement for others.[10] Meals and emotional stress exacerbate abdominal pain for some patients.[11]

Patients with IBS often report altered bowel movements, such as diarrhea, constipation, alternating diarrhea and constipation, or predominantly normal bowel movements with occasional diarrhea or constipation. The Bristol stool scale (**Fig. 1**) can help patients to identify which type of stool is most frequently observed in their bowel movements.

Patients with IBS and diarrhea-predominant symptoms describe frequent soft stools with an appearance of soft blobs, fluffy pieces, or watery liquid stools (type 5–7 on the Bristol stool scale). Bowel movements occur throughout the day and are often associated with meals. Approximately half of patients with IBS report mucus discharge with stools.[12] Patients with IBS and constipation report hard stools with infrequent bowel movements (type 1–2 on the Bristol stool scale). These patients also commonly complain of incomplete evacuation and tenesmus. Women with IBS are more prone to have constipation.[11]

CLASSIFICATION OF IRRITABLE BOWEL SYNDROME

The Rome criteria were established by functional bowel disease experts to help better manage patients with abdominal symptoms consistent with IBS. Using this classification, IBS is classified according to the predominant stool pattern[13]:

1. IBS with predominant constipation (IBS-C); greater than 25% hard stools and less than 25% loose stools
2. IBS with predominant diarrhea (IBS-D): greater than 25% loose stools and less than 25% hard stools
3. IBS with mixed bowel habits (IBS-M): greater than 25% loose stools and greater than 25% hard stools
4. IBS unclassified (IBS-U): less than 25% loose stools and less than 25% hard stools

RED FLAG SYMPTOMS

IBS symptoms may be nonspecific, but during evaluation of symptoms, it is important to ask about "red flag" symptoms. These are not considered symptoms of IBS and always require further evaluation. The red flag symptoms include the following[14]:

- Age older than 50
- Nocturnal symptoms, especially diarrhea
- Bloody stool
- Fever
- Weight loss
- Abnormal laboratory tests (including anemia, elevated inflammatory markers)
- Family history of inflammatory bowel disease or colon cancer

The Bristol Stool Form Scale

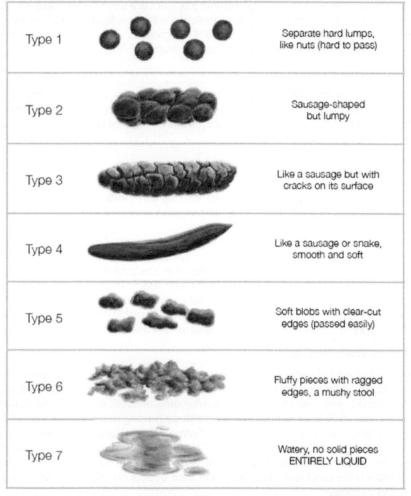

Type 1		Separate hard lumps, like nuts (hard to pass)
Type 2		Sausage-shaped but lumpy
Type 3		Like a sausage but with cracks on its surface
Type 4		Like a sausage or snake, smooth and soft
Type 5		Soft blobs with clear-cut edges (passed easily)
Type 6		Fluffy pieces with ragged edges, a mushy stool
Type 7		Watery, no solid pieces ENTIRELY LIQUID

Fig. 1. The Bristol stool scale provides a visual tool for patients to classify their stool consistency ranging from firm balls (type 1) to thin liquid (type 7). (Distributed with the kind permission of Dr K. W. Heaton; formerly reader in medicine at the University of Bristol. Reproduced as a service to the medical profession by Norgine Ltd. ©2017 Norgine group of companies.)

PATHOPHYSIOLOGY OF IRRITABLE BOWEL SYNDROME

IBS is no longer regarded as an idiopathic bowel dysfunction that originates exclusively from psychological stress. The pathophysiology of IBS is complex and is due to a combination of several factors. No single specific cause for this disorder has been identified.[15] There are multiple areas of ongoing research into the underlying etiology of IBS, which include research on alterations in gastrointestinal motility, visceral hypersensitivity and neuro-enteric dysregulation, the role of inflammation, bile acids, alterations in fecal flora, bacterial overgrowth, the microbiome, food sensitivity, and genetic predisposition.

Alterations in Gastrointestinal Motility

Motility abnormalities of the gastrointestinal (GI) tract are seen in some but not all patients with IBS. Approximately 25% of patients with constipation-predominant IBS have slow colonic transit and 15% to 45% of patients with diarrhea-predominant IBS were noted to have acceleration of colonic transit.[16,17]

Visceral Hypersensitivity

It was first demonstrated in 1973 that patients with IBS experienced an increased pain response to rectal balloon distension compared with healthy individuals.[18] Another study showed that rectal distension in patients with IBS increased cerebral cortical activity more than in controls.[19]

Food Hypersensitivity

Although well-defined food allergies are not common in patients with IBS, exacerbation of IBS symptoms has been observed with certain foods, particularly in patients with diarrhea-predominant IBS. These are termed food sensitivities, and are not true immunoglobulin (Ig)E-mediated food allergies.

IBS symptoms also may be increased with high-fat meals. One study examined the effect of a fat-rich liquid meal of 600 kcal on visceral perception in subjects with IBS and healthy controls. The study demonstrated that postprandial, but not fasting, pain scores were significantly elevated in patients with IBS.[20] In another study examining the correlation between meals and IBS, rectal sensitivity increased significantly in patients with IBS at 30 and 60 minutes after a high-fat meal.[21] These studies suggest a role for dietary fat content in IBS-related discomfort and pain.

Fecal Short-Chain Fatty Acids

Fecal short-chain fatty acids (SCFAs) may also play a role in IBS symptoms, as they are increased in stool from patients with diarrhea-predominant IBS.[22] SCFAs stimulate colonic transit and motility through intraluminal release of 5-hydroxytryptamine (5-HT)[23] in rats. SCFAs also initiate high-amplitude propagated contractions in the colon, propelling colonic content rapidly.[24] Fermentable oligosaccharides, disaccharides, monosaccharides, and polyols (FODMAPs), which are found in a variety of foods, are poorly absorbed in the small intestine and may induce symptoms of IBS[25] through the production of SCFAs and their effects on colonic motility, contractions, and secretion.

Gluten

The role of gluten in IBS has been of interest to gastroenterology researchers and the public. A randomized, placebo-controlled trial involving patients who previously reported intolerance to gluten and a response to its withdrawal confirmed that gluten was associated with symptoms of IBS.[26] In a recent randomized controlled trial (RCT) of a gluten-containing diet versus a gluten-free diet in patients with IBS-D, participants ingesting gluten had increased stool frequency, increased bowel permeability, and reduced messenger RNA expression of tight-junction proteins in the bowel mucosa.[27] In another study of patients with IBS with diarrhea, but without celiac disease, researchers found that dietary gluten altered small intestinal permeability and had a greater effect on bowel movement frequency in patients who were HLA-DQ2/8 positive compared with those who were HLA-DQ2/8 negative.[28]

Fructose

Fructose intake can also contribute to symptoms of IBS. Fructose is a 6-carbon monosaccharide. It is naturally present in a variety of foods, such as fruits, vegetables, and honey. It is also enzymatically produced from corn as high-fructose corn syrup, which is a common food sweetener found in soft drinks and condiments. Approximately one-third of patients with suspected IBS have fructose malabsorption and dietary fructose intolerance.[9] Malabsorption of fructose leads to water influx into the lumen due to osmotic pressure. This, in turn, results in rapid propulsion of bowel contents into the colon. Unabsorbed fructose is fermented by colonic bacteria, which results in the production of SCFAs, hydrogen, carbon dioxide, and trace gases. This can result in symptoms including abdominal pain, excessive gas, and bloating.[29]

Bile Acids

A systematic review of the literature suggested that bile acid malabsorption accounts for approximately 30% of cases of IBS-D.[30] In another study, approximately 25% of patients with IBS-D had an elevated 48-hour total fecal bile acid excretion compared with IBS-C. In this study, 40% of patients with IBS-D showed elevated bile acid synthesis (as measured by the fasting concentration of a bile acid precursor) compared with healthy controls and patients with IBS-C.[31]

Microbiota

The precise role of the fecal or mucosal microbiome in IBS is unclear. Studies of the mucosa-associated microbiota in patients with IBS-D have shown increases in *Bacteroides* and *Clostridia* and a reduction in bifidobacteria.[32] A negative relationship between the fecal abundance of bifidobacteria and pain score in IBS has been reported.[32,33] The role of the microbiome in IBS symptoms is suggested by meta-analysis data showing the efficacy of probiotics,[34] particularly for abdominal pain and bloating. In addition, a probiotic mixture has been shown to slow colonic transit in patients with IBS-D, suggesting that the gut microbiome may have a role in the symptoms of IBS.[35]

Small Intestinal Bacterial Overgrowth

Small intestinal bacterial overgrowth (SIBO) also has been investigated as a contributor to IBS. Several studies have shown that some patients with IBS, especially patients with IBS-D, have an abnormal lactulose breath test (elevated breath hydrogen), suggestive of SIBO. These same patients showed improvement in pain and diarrhea after eradication of bacterial overgrowth.[36,37] In addition to elevated breath hydrogen, increased methane production during lactulose breath testing has been seen in some patients with IBS-C.[38]

Inflammation

Mucosal inflammation has been associated with increased intestinal permeability and may play a role in IBS. In some patients with IBS, there are increased levels of T lymphocytes, and in some cases, mast cells in the rectal mucosa.[39] These data, in addition to the epidemiologic and clinical observations seen in patients with postinfectious IBS,[40] support a role of immune activation and altered bowel barrier function in a subgroup of patients with IBS. Genetic susceptibility may confer a predisposition to immune activation in a subset of patients with IBS.

Genetic

Genetic factors may play a role in development of IBS. Some areas of research include genetic differences in predisposition to inflammation, bile acid synthesis, and intestinal secretion.

DIAGNOSIS OF IRRITABLE BOWEL SYNDROME

Diagnosis of IBS is made based on clinical symptoms that meet the diagnostic criteria and a basic evaluation to exclude other organic diseases that mimic the symptoms of IBS. Due to the absence of specific blood test, markers, and imaging studies that can help diagnose IBS, multiple definitions and diagnostic criteria have been used to diagnose IBS. The Rome consensus criteria were established in 1989 to help guide clinicians in understanding IBS. The most recent criteria, the Rome IV criteria, were released in May of 2016.[13]

ROME IV

IBS is defined as recurrent abdominal pain for at least 1 day per week in the past 3 months, associated with 2 or more of the following criteria[13]:

- Related to defecation
- Associated with a change in stool frequency
- Associated with a change in stool form

CLINICAL EVALUATION
History and Physical Examination

This is the most important part of the evaluation because the diagnosis of IBS is predominantly based on symptoms. A complete history and physical can identify alarm symptoms, and help to exclude conditions that might mimic the symptoms of IBS, such as inflammatory bowel disease, celiac disease, or malignancy. Specific features of the medical history that may be helpful include family history, medications, prior history of viral or bacterial gastrointestinal infection, and symptoms related to fatty meals or gluten. A thorough physical examination in the average patient with IBS would typically be unrevealing. Findings such as dermatitis, rebound, guarding, point tenderness, or blood in stool, joint dysfunction, or arthritis should prompt an appropriate workup for other causes of GI symptoms. Any patient presenting with red flag/alarm symptoms should undergo further evaluation.

Laboratory Tests

A complete blood count helps to exclude anemia. Anemia, including iron deficiency anemia, is not expected with IBS and requires further workup to identify the underlying disorder. For patients with IBS-D, stool testing can be considered. Ova and parasite testing, particularly if there is prior exposure to lake or spring water, can be performed to look for infection. Inflammatory markers such as C-reactive protein or fecal lactoferrin can assess for inflammatory bowel disease. Celiac serologies (tissue transglutaminase IgA) can be checked to exclude celiac disease from the differential.

DIFFERENTIAL DIAGNOSIS

The differential diagnosis of IBS is broad. A good history and physical with a few laboratory tests can help exclude celiac disease, inflammatory bowel disease, microscopic colitis, post-cholecystectomy bile acid diarrhea, and SIBO. Patients with

IBS-C also can have pelvic floor dysfunction or colonic transit disorders. If treatment fails to improve symptoms, then additional evaluation may be required. A rectal examination can help to identify patients who also have dyssynergia or pelvic floor problems.

MANAGEMENT

Management of IBS can include dietary modification, medications, and mind-body treatments.

Dietary Intervention

Diet modification is one of the most commonly used interventions for patients with IBS.[41] A careful dietary history might suggest symptoms related to specific foods.

Commonly Recommended Dietary Modifications

Diet low in fermentable oligosaccharides, disaccharides, monosaccharides, and polyols

The low-FODMAP diet has been studied in patients with IBS. The acronym FODMAP describes the oligosaccharides fructans and galacto-oligosaccharides present in wheat, rye, onions, garlic, and legumes; the disaccharide lactose present in milk and yogurt; the monosaccharide fructose (when consumed in excess of glucose) present in honey, apples, pears, and high-fructose corn syrup; and polyols including sorbitol and mannitol present in apples, pears, stone fruit, and many artificially sweetened gums and confectionary.[42] The efficacy of the elimination phase of the low-FODMAP diet for overall GI symptom relief in adult patients with IBS has been examined in RCTs; a blinded, randomized, rechallenge study; and observational studies. These studies have shown that 50% to 86% of patients have a clinically meaningful response to the low-FODMAP diet.[43]

Fructans and galacto-oligosaccharides have prebiotic actions in the gastrointestinal tract. Their restriction, in the setting of the low-FODMAP diet, may lead to a reduction in beneficial bacteria. For this reason, it is generally recommended to administer the low-FODMAP diet in 2 phases. The first phase is to assess the patient's degree of benefit from the diet. This is best achieved through an initial phase of strict elimination of foods high in FODMAPs, generally of 6 to 8 weeks' duration, guided by a specialist dietician. After finishing the initial 6 to 8 weeks of the low-FODMAP diet, a follow-up consultation with a dietician is indicated. The patient's diet is then liberalized in a stepwise fashion to determine the type and amount of FODMAPs that can be tolerated. This second phase tailors the low-FODMAP diet to each patient to ensure that unnecessary dietary restriction is minimized and maximum variety in the diet is achieved, while still maintaining a satisfactory level of symptom control.[42]

High-fiber diet

Fiber supplementation has traditionally been recommended for patients with IBS and has received much attention; however, most research studies examining the role of fiber in treatment of IBS have shown no clear difference over placebo.[44]

Gas-producing foods

For patients with IBS, some benefit may occur from reducing gas-producing foods. These include beans, onions, celery, carrots, raisins, bananas, apricots, prunes, Brussels sprouts, wheat germ, pretzels, and bagels. Reduction in consumption of these foods may reduce gas formation, bloating, and flatulence. This diet is less restrictive than the FODMAP diet.

Dietary Recommendations for Selected Cases

Gluten-free diet

Evidence to support gluten avoidance in patients with nonceliac gluten sensitivity (NCGS) has been conflicting. In a randomized double-blind crossover trial, 59 patients with NCGS on a gluten-free diet were assigned to receive gluten (without fructan), fructan (without gluten), or placebo for 7 days.[45] GI symptom rating scores and bloating were higher with fructan than with gluten. There was no difference in symptom scores between gluten and placebo groups. This study suggests that symptomatic improvement with a gluten-free diet in such patients may not be due to removal of the gluten protein, but due to reduced exposure to fructan, which foods with gluten often contain.

A role for the low-FODMAP diet in people with NCGS was recently suggested in a double-blinded placebo-controlled crossover trial in patients with self-reported NCGS.[46] This study showed that gluten did not induce any specific GI symptoms in the 37 participants; however, the provision of a low-FODMAP diet reduced symptoms in all 37 participants, leading to greater symptom improvement than following a gluten-free diet ($P<.001$).

Lactose-free diet

There is no evidence to suggest that the incidence of lactose malabsorption is higher in patients with IBS. Some studies have shown that patients with IBS and lactose intolerance have an exaggerated symptom response to lactose ingestion.[47] If a dietary history suggests lactose malabsorption, substantial relief of symptoms can be achieved with lactase enzyme supplementation during mealtimes.

Less Frequently Used Diets in Clinical Practice

Elimination diet

More intensive elimination diets have been described, and in one small study of 25 patients, improvement of IBS symptoms was seen. The strict elimination diet consisted of distilled or spring water, 1 meat, and 1 fruit for a week. Two-thirds of patients who completed this diet noted symptom improvement followed by a worsening of symptoms when suspect foods were reintroduced.[48,49] Extreme diets are not ideal for long-term use and may cause nutritional deficiencies. It is not recommended to follow overly restrictive diets to manage IBS symptoms.

Immunoglobulin G–related food symptoms

One study examined the potential role of IgG-related food responses as a guide for symptom management. Patients with IBS in this 12-week randomized, blinded trial received a diet excluding foods to which they had increased IgG antibodies. With these dietary changes, the study patients showed improvement in IBS symptoms.[48] At this time, there is insufficient evidence to support routine food allergy testing in patients with IBS. No GI society endorses IgG testing to guide food elimination diets for IBS outside of a research setting. It is reasonable to avoid allergens in susceptible patients, provided this would not substantially impair their dietary intake.

Pharmacotherapy Targeted to Irritable Bowel Syndrome Symptoms

In addition to dietary modification, medications are helpful in managing IBS symptoms. Choice of medication will depend on the symptoms reported by the patient (**Table 1**).

Abdominal pain

Tricyclic antidepressants For the treatment of abdominal pain in IBS, antidepressants have shown benefit in clinical studies and ideally should be started at low doses. The initial dose should be adjusted based on tolerance and response. Tricyclic antidepressants (TCAs) can slow the GI transit time due to their anticholinergic effect, which may be particularly helpful in IBS-D. A systematic review showed a modest improvement in global relief and abdominal pain in patients treated with TCAs, although the overall body of evidence was of low quality. TCAs are a low-cost option for treatment of symptoms in patients with IBS; however, they should be used with caution in patients at risk for prolongation of the QT interval.[50]

Antispasmodics The antispasmodics hyoscyamine, dicyclomine, and peppermint oil have also been studied in IBS. A meta-analysis showed significant improvement in IBS-related global symptoms with antispasmodics. Studies also showed modest improvement in abdominal pain symptoms with minimal risk of adverse effects.[50] In another meta-analysis of 9 randomized placebo-controlled trials including 726 patients, peppermint oil was found to be significantly superior to placebo for global improvement of IBS symptoms and improvement in abdominal pain.[51]

Selective serotonin reuptake inhibitors

Selective serotonin reuptake inhibitors (SSRIs) have been extensively studied in IBS, and results have been lackluster compared with TCAs. Pooled estimates from 5 RCTs show no improvement in global relief of symptoms. In addition, 4 RCTs showed no improvement in abdominal pain. However, the risk of important adverse effects is minimal. The American Gastroenterological Association recommends against using SSRIs as primary therapy for patients with IBS, but as some studies did show a benefit, they can still be considered as an option for treatment. Patients with depression do not need to discontinue SSRI therapy to improve IBS symptoms.[50]

Diarrhea

Rifaximin Rifaximin is an oral nonsystemic GI-targeted antibiotic that has in vitro activity against a variety of gram-negative and gram-positive bacteria.[52] Pooled data from several studies of rifaximin in IBS showed a small, but beneficial, effect of rifaximin with improvement in abdominal pain and stool consistency. Three RCTs demonstrated an improvement in IBS-related global symptoms. Additionally, these studies showed small improvements in abdominal pain and bloating. Symptom relief was reported, but few studies have documented sustained relief for all patients with IBS.[50] It is important to note that although side effects were minimal, the cost of treatment may be quite high.

Loperamide Loperamide is a peripherally acting μ-opioid receptor agonist. This is the only antidiarrheal agent evaluated in randomized trials in patients with IBS-D. Data investigating the use of loperamide specifically for the treatment of patients with IBS-D, as opposed to symptomatic relief of diarrhea for other disease states, is very limited. Two older RCTs that in the aggregate enrolled 42 patients failed to show a significant benefit in global relief of IBS-related symptoms. However, the quality of evidence from these trials was very low due to methodological concerns. There is a large body of indirect evidence from a variety of other settings that shows the efficacy of loperamide in reducing stool frequency. Therefore, because of low cost, wide availability, and minimal adverse effects, loperamide can be viewed as a useful adjunct to other IBS-D therapies.[50]

Bile acid sequestrants Bile acid sequestrants, such as cholestyramine, colestipol, and colesevelam, can be used to manage IBS-D. Bile acid agents bind to luminal bile acids, impeding reabsorption, and reducing stimulation of colonic transit. These agents may be effective in patients with IBS-D, as bile acid diarrhea is due to either increased bile acid synthesis or impaired reabsorption.[53] In an open-label trial, colesevelam showed evidence of intraluminal binding of bile acids and improved stool consistency in patients with IBS-D.[54] Bile acid sequestrants can be associated with GI side effects, including bloating, flatulence, abdominal discomfort, and constipation.

Alosetron Alosetron is a 5-hydroxytryptamine-3 receptor antagonist. Based on pooled data from multiple RCTs, patients treated with alosetron had improvement in abdominal pain and IBS-related global symptoms. However, postmarketing data from an observational study suggested that idiopathic, non–dose-dependent ischemic colitis could occur with use (approximately 1 case/1000 patient-years). The drug was voluntarily withdrawn from the market and subsequently reintroduced only under a physician-based risk management program.[50] Alosetron is used only for the treatment of severe diarrhea-predominant IBS lasting for at least 6 months in women who failed to respond to other treatments. Good candidates for this medication should have few risk factors for ischemic disease.

Eluxadoline Eluxadoline is a mu-opioid receptor agonist and a delta-opioid receptor antagonist. Eluxadoline has been approved for treatment of IBS-D and can dramatically reduce bowel movement frequency and improve consistency. It is contraindicated in patients with history of biliary disease, severe liver disease (Child-Pugh Class C), pancreatitis, and heavy alcohol use. It is also contraindicated in patients without a gallbladder due to an increased incidence of severe acute pancreatitis noted in postmarketing surveillance.[55]

Constipation
Laxatives are effective in increasing the frequency of bowel movements, and therefore a simple way to manage the constipation symptom of IBS-C.

Polyethylene glycol laxatives A polyethylene glycol (PEG) laxative is an inexpensive laxative that is easily tolerated by patients. It is mainly used in IBS-C to improve constipation. There are several trials examining the use of PEG laxatives in patients with chronic constipation; however, there is only one RCT evaluating the use of PEG solution for treating patients with IBS-C. This 4-week trial did not show a measurable effect of PEG laxatives on IBS-related global symptom scores.[50]

Linaclotide Linaclotide is a guanylate cyclase C receptor agonist that increases luminal chloride and fluid secretion through the generation of cyclic guanosine monophosphate. Linaclotide is used for the treatment of IBS-C at a dosage of 290 µg daily. Two randomized trials of linaclotide in patients with IBS-C showed a modest beneficial effect with a combined improvement in abdominal pain and an increase in the number of complete spontaneous bowel movements and improvement in global symptoms. Diarrhea leading to treatment discontinuation occurred in a small percentage of treated patients.[50]

Lubiprostone Lubiprostone is a chloride channel activator that triggers intestinal chloride secretion and sodium and fluid transit into the lumen. It is used for the treatment of IBS-C at a dosage of 8 µg twice daily. Dosages can be escalated to 16 and 24 µg twice daily in patients who do not respond completely to lower dosages. Two randomized trials of lubiprostone were performed in patients with IBS-C. Most patients were women, and the placebo response in the studies was far lower than expected.[56] In these 2 multicenter, placebo-controlled trials, 1154 adults with IBS and constipation were randomly assigned to lubiprostone (8 μg twice daily) or placebo for 12 weeks. Patients randomized to lubiprostone were significantly more likely to achieve an overall symptom response (18% vs 10%). Serious adverse events were similar to placebo. The most common adverse event was nausea (8% vs 4%). A follow-up open-label study that included 522 patients demonstrated that benefits of lubiprostone persisted or increased at 52 weeks. There are 2 RCTs of 12 weeks' duration examining the effectiveness of lubiprostone for global symptom relief in patients with IBS-C, with a pooled effect estimate showing a small improvement in global symptoms of IBS. There were few adverse effects from using lubiprostone.[50]

Plecanatide Plecanatide is a novel agent affecting guanylate cyclase recently approved by the Food and Drug Administration for management of IBS-C. This medication promotes bowel transit and adds water to soften the stool as it passes through the gut. A recent study demonstrated the efficacy and safety of plecanatide for both pain and constipation symptoms.[57]

Mind-body techniques
Hypnotherapy Gut-directed hypnotherapy for IBS has been tested in RCTs, which have shown efficacy in IBS cohorts.[58] A recent randomized clinical trial compared the short-term and long-term efficacy of gut-directed hypnotherapy and the low-FODMAP diet and found similar durable effects for the relief of GI symptoms.[59] Seventy-four patients were randomly allocated to receive treatment via hypnotherapy (n = 25), diet (n = 24), or both (n = 25). Clinically significant improvements in overall GI symptoms were observed from baseline to week 6 in 72%, 71%, and 73% of patients, respectively. This improvement persisted 6 months posttreatment in 74%, 82%, and 54% of patients, leading the researchers to conclude that gut-directed hypnotherapy showed efficacy similar to the low-FODMAP diet, but no additional benefit when these modalities were combined. Although IBS quality of life was significantly improved across all groups, hypnotherapy resulted in superior improvements in psychological indices.

Acupuncture Several studies have confirmed that acupuncture is effective treatment for IBS, as it can regulate the brain-gut axis and improve visceral hyperactivity.[60] Electro-acupuncture showed good therapeutic effect on C-IBS abdominal pain and bloating. It also improved defecation frequency, constipation, difficulty in defecation, and other main GI symptoms. Electro-acupuncture also alleviated depression, anxiety, and other psychological symptoms, and also affected brain-related functional areas.[61]

Cognitive behavioral therapy Cognitive behavioral therapy (CBT) has also been studied in patients with IBS. In an RCT, it was found that a home-based version of CBT produced significant and long-term GI symptom improvement for patients with IBS compared with IBS education alone.[62]

OVERALL STRATEGY FOR IRRITABLE BOWEL SYNDROME MANAGEMENT

The main strategy for management of symptoms in IBS is to improve each symptom, starting with the symptom that is most bothersome to the patient. It is critical to form a therapeutic alliance with the patient, building trust and confidence in a collaborative approach. A therapeutic relationship begins with good communication, including caring language in the visit, eye contact, and providing verbal reassurance that you as a diagnostician will continue to work with the patient over time until the symptoms improve. For mild IBS symptoms, less intensive strategies, such as healthy diet (avoiding junk food), improved quality of sleep, and relaxation strategies to avoid anxiety and stress may be sufficient. A short dietary intervention with low-FODMAP foods can be followed by an organized reintroduction of foods, to quantify the effect of trigger foods on symptoms. A nutritionist can be very helpful and there are many online dietary resources to help guide patients as well. A rational approach to long-term dietary change is important. For moderate IBS with persistent symptoms, gut-directed medications also can be helpful. For diarrhea-predominant symptoms, loperamide, rifaximin, or bile acid binding agents can be trialed. For pain-predominant symptoms, tricyclic antidepressants or SSRIs can be used. For constipation-predominant symptoms, chloride channel and guanylate cyclase agents can be considered, such as lubiprostone, linaclotide, and plecanatide. For more severe daily symptoms that are troublesome and persistent, some patients may require combination therapy, including dietary modification, medications, and psychological interventions, such as CBT to help manage symptoms. The combination of different types of therapy and a strong therapeutic alliance with the patient is a winning strategy for IBS symptom control.

Table 1
Medication strategies for symptom management in irritable bowel syndrome

Symptom	Medication Strategy
Diarrhea-focused symptoms	Loperamide 2 mg every few hours as needed, no more than 8 doses per day
	Cholestyramine 9 g twice or thrice daily
	Colestipol 2 g daily or twice daily
	Colesevelam 625 mg daily or twice daily as tolerated
	Probiotics multiple formulations
	Rifaximin 550 mg by mouth thrice daily for 14 d
	Alosetron 0.5 mg to 1 mg daily as tolerated
	Ondansetron 4–8 mg 3 times daily
	Eluxadoline 100 mg twice daily as tolerated
Constipation-focused symptoms	Psyllium 30 g daily in divided doses
	Polyethylene glycol agents 17 g daily or twice daily
	Lubiprostone 8 µg twice daily, titrate to 24 µg twice daily as tolerated
	Linaclotide 290 µg daily, although 145-µg and 72-µg dosing also available if not tolerated
	Plecanatide 3 mg daily
Abdominal pain–focused symptoms	Dicyclomine 10 mg daily to 4 times daily, titrate up to 20 mg if needed
	Peppermint oil 250–750 mg twice daily or thrice daily
	Desipramine 25–100 mg nightly
	Amitriptyline 10–50 mg nightly
	Paroxetine 10–40 mg daily
	Sertraline 25–100 mg daily
	Citalopram 10–40 mg daily
	Linaclotide, alosetron, lubiprostone, and plecanatide show improvement in pain relief and also can be used for pain-predominant symptoms

REFERENCES

1. Lacy BE, Mearin F, Chang L, et al. Bowel disorders. Gastroenterology 2016;150: 1393–407.

2. Longstreth GF, Thompson WG, Chey WD, et al. Functional bowel disorders. Gastroenterology 2006;130:1480–91.

3. Camilleri M, Choi MG. Review article: irritable bowel syndrome. Aliment Pharmacol Ther 1997;11(1):3–15.

4. Everhart JE, Renault PF. Irritable bowel syndrome in office-based practice in the United States. Gastroenterology 1991;100(4):998.

5. Sayuk GS, Wolf R, Chang L. Comparison of symptoms, healthcare utilization, and treatment in diagnosed and undiagnosed individuals with diarrhea-predominant irritable bowel syndrome. Am J Gastroenterol 2017;112(6):892.

6. Choung RS, Locke GR 3rd. Epidemiology of IBS. Gastroenterol Clin North Am 2011;40:1–10.

7. Lovell RM, Ford AC. Global prevalence of and risk factors for irritable bowel syndrome: a meta-analysis. Clin Gastroenterol Hepatol 2012;10:712–21.e4.

8. Hungin APS, Chang L, Locke GR, et al. Irritable bowel syndrome in the United States: prevalence, symptom patterns and impact. Aliment Pharmacol Ther 2005;21:1365–75.

9. Ikechi R, Fischer B, DeSipio J, et al. Irritable bowel syndrome: clinical manifestations, dietary influences, and management. Healthcare (Basel) 2017;5(2):21.

10. Walter SA, Ragnarsson G, Bodemar G. New criteria for irritable bowel syndrome based on prospective symptom evaluation. Am J Gastroenterol 2005;100(11):2598–9.

11. Ragnarsson G, Bodemar G. Pain is temporally related to eating but not to defaecation in the irritable bowel syndrome (IBS). Patients' description of diarrhea, constipation and symptom variation during a prospective 6-week study. Eur J Gastroenterol Hepatol 1998;10(5):415–21.

12. Manning AP, Thompson WG, Heaton KW, et al. Towards positive diagnosis of the irritable bowel. Br Med J 1978;2(6138):653.

13. Simren M, Olafur S, Palsson, et al. Update on Rome IV criteria for colorectal disorders: implications for clinical practice. Curr Gastroenterol Rep 2017;19:15.

14. Brandt LJ, Chey WD, Foxx-Orenstein AE, et al. An evidence-based position statement on the management of irritable bowel syndrome. American College of Gastroenterology Task Force on Irritable Bowel Syndrome. Am J Gastroenterol 2009;104(Suppl 1):S1.

15. Camilleri M. Peripheral mechanisms in irritable bowel syndrome. N Engl J Med 2012;367(17):1626–35.

16. Camilleri M, McKinzie S, Busciglio I, et al. Prospective study of motor, sensory, psychologic, and autonomic functions in patients with irritable bowel syndrome. Clin Gastroenterol Hepatol 2008;6:772–81.

17. Törnblom H, Van Oudenhove L, Sadik R, et al. Colonic transit time and IBS symptoms: what's the link? Am J Gastroenterol 2012;107:754–60.

18. Ritchie J. Pain from distension of the pelvic colon by inflating a balloon in the irritable colon syndrome. Gut 1973;14:125–32.

19. Lawal A, Kern M, Sidhu H, et al. Novel evidence for hypersensitivity of visceral sensory neural circuitry in irritable bowel syndrome patients. Gastroenterology 2006;130(1):26.

20. van der Veek PPJ, Steenvoorden J, Steens PJ, et al. Recto-colonic reflex is impaired in patients with irritable bowel syndrome. Neurogastroenterol Motil 2007;19(8):653–9.

21. Simren M, Agerforz P, Björnsson S, et al. Nutrient-dependent enhancement of rectal sensitivity in irritable bowel syndrome (IBS). Neurogastroenterol Motil 2007;19(1):20–9.

22. Treem WR, Ahsan N, Kastoff G, et al. Fecal short-chain fatty acids in patients with diarrhea-predominant irritable bowel syndrome: in vitro studies of carbohydrate fermentation. J Pediatr Gastroenterol Nutr 1996;23:280–6.
23. Fukumoto S, Tatewaki M, Yamada T, et al. Short-chain fatty acids stimulate colonic transit via intraluminal 5-HT release in rats. Am J Physiol Regul Integr Comp Physiol 2003;284:R1269–76.
24. Kamath PS, Hoepfner MT, Phillips SF. Short-chain fatty acids stimulate motility of the canine ileum. Am J Physiol 1987;253:G427–33.
25. Shepherd SJ, Parker FC, Muir JG, et al. Dietary triggers of abdominal symptoms in patients with irritable bowel syndrome: randomized, placebo-controlled evidence. Clin Gastroenterol Hepatol 2008;6:765–71.
26. Biesiekierski JR, Newnham ED, Irving PM, et al. Gluten causes gastrointestinal symptoms in subjects without celiac disease: a double-blind randomized placebo-controlled trial. Am J Gastroenterol 2011;106:508–14.
27. Camilleri M, Vazquez-Roque MI, Carlson P, et al. Randomized trial of gluten-free diet in IBS-diarrhea: effect on small bowel and colonic morphology and barrier function. Neurogastroenterol Motil 2012;24:23.
28. Vazquez-Roque MI, Camilleri M, Smyrk T, et al. A controlled trial of gluten-free diet in patients with irritable bowel syndrome-diarrhea: effects on bowel frequency and intestinal function. Gastroenterology 2013;144(5):903–11.e3.
29. DiNicolantonio JJ, Lucan SC. Is fructose malabsorption a cause of irritable bowel syndrome? Med Hypotheses 2015;85:295–7.
30. Wedlake L, A'Hern R, Russell D, et al. Systematic review: the prevalence of idiopathic bile acid malabsorption as diagnosed by SeHCAT scanning in patients with diarrhoea-predominant irritable bowel syndrome. Aliment Pharmacol Ther 2009;30:707–17.
31. Wong BS, Camilleri M, Carlson P, et al. Increased bile acid biosynthesis is associated with irritable bowel syndrome with diarrhea. Clin Gastroenterol Hepatol 2012;10:1009–15.
32. Parkes GC, Rayment NB, Hudspith BN, et al. Distinct microbial populations exist in the mucosa-associated microbiota of sub-groups of irritable bowel syndrome. Neurogastroenterol Motil 2012;24:31–9.
33. Rajilic-Sotjanovic M, Biagi E, Heilig HG, et al. Global and deep molecular analysis of microbiota signatures in faecal samples from patients with irritable bowel syndrome. Gastroenterology 2011;141:1737–801.
34. Moayyedi P, Ford AC, Talley NJ, et al. The efficacy of probiotics in the treatment of irritable bowel syndrome: a systematic review. Gut 2010;59:325–32.
35. Kim HJ, Camilleri M, McKinzie S, et al. A randomized, controlled trial of a probiotic, VSL#3, on gut transit and symptoms in diarrhea-predominant irritable bowel syndrome. Aliment Pharmacol Ther 2003;17:895–904.
36. Pimentel M, Chow EJ, Lin HC. Normalization of lactulose breath testing correlates with symptom improvement in irritable bowel syndrome. a double-blind, randomized, placebo-controlled study. Am J Gastroenterol 2003;98(2):412.
37. Pimentel M, Chow EJ, Lin HC. Eradication of small intestinal bacterial overgrowth reduces symptoms of irritable bowel syndrome. Am J Gastroenterol 2000;95(12):3503.
38. Chatterjee S, Park S, Low K, et al. The degree of breath methane production in IBS correlates with the severity of constipation. Am J Gastroenterol 2007;102(4):837.
39. Spiller RC, Jenkins D, Thornley JP, et al. Increased rectal mucosal enteroendocrine cells, T lymphocytes, and increased gut permeability following acute

Campylobacter enteritis and in post-dysenteric irritable bowel syndrome. Gut 2000;47:804–11.

40. Spiller R, Garsed K. Postinfectious irritable bowel syndrome. Gastroenterology 2009;136:1979–88.

41. Lacy BE. The science, evidence, and practice of dietary interventions in irritable bowel syndrome. Clin Gastroenterol Hepatol 2015;13:1899–906.

42. Shepherd SJ, Lomer MCE, Gibson PR. Short-chain carbohydrates and & functional gastrointestinal disorders. Am J Gastroenterol 2013;108:707–17.

43. Hill P, Muir JG, Gibson PR. Controversies and recent developments of the low-FODMAP diet. Gastroenterol Hepatol (N Y) 2017;13(1):36–45.

44. Eswaran S, Muir J, Chey WD. Fiber and functional gastrointestinal disorders. Am J Gastroenterol 2013;108:718–27.

45. Skodje GI, Sarna VK, Minelle IH, et al. Fructan, rather than gluten, induces symptoms in patients with self-reported non-celiac gluten sensitivity. Gastroenterology 2018;154(3):529.

46. Biesiekierski JR, Peters SL, Newnham ED, et al. No effects of gluten in patients with self-reported nonceliac gluten sensitivity after dietary reduction of fermentable, poorly absorbed, short-chain carbohydrates. Gastroenterology 2013;145:320–8.

47. Zhu Y, Zheng X, Cong Y, et al. Bloating and distention in irritable bowel syndrome: the role of gas production and visceral sensation after lactose ingestion in a population with lactase deficiency. Am J Gastroenterol 2013;108(9):1516.

48. Jones VA, Mclaughlan P, Shorthouse M, et al. Food intolerance: a major factor in the pathogenesis of irritable bowel syndrome. Lancet 1982;2:1115–7.

49. Atkinson W, Sheldon TA, Shaath N, et al. Food elimination based on IgG antibodies in irritable bowel syndrome: a randomised controlled trial. Gut 2004;53:1459–64.

50. Weinberg DS, Smalley W, Heidelbaugh JJ, et al. American Gastroenterological Association institute guideline on the pharmacological management of irritable bowel syndrome. Gastroenterology 2014;147:1146–8.

51. Khanna R, MacDonald JK, Levesque BG. Peppermint oil for the treatment of irritable bowel syndrome. A systematic review and meta-analysis. J Clin Gastroenterol 2014;48(6):505–12.

52. Jiang ZD, DuPont HL. Rifaximin: in vitro and in vivo antibacterial activity—a review. Chemotherapy 2005;51:67–72.

53. Shin A, Camilleri M, Vijayvargiya P, et al. Bowel functions, fecal unconjugated primary and secondary bile acids, and colonic transit in patients with irritable bowel syndrome. Clin Gastroenterol Hepatol 2013;11:1270–5.e1.

54. Camilleri M, Acosta A, Busciglio I, et al. Effect of colesevelam on faecal bile acids and bowel functions in diarrhoea-predominant irritable bowel syndrome. Aliment Pharmacol Ther 2015;41:438–48.

55. Available at: https://www.fda.gov/Drugs/DrugSafety/ucm546154.htm. Accessed June 13, 2018.

56. Drossman DA, Chey WD, Johanson JF, et al. Clinical trial: lubiprostone in patients with constipation-associated irritable bowel syndrome—results of two randomized, placebo-controlled studies. Aliment Pharmacol Ther 2009;29(3):329.

57. Brenner DM, Fogel R, Dorn SD, et al. Efficacy, safety, and tolerability of plecanatide in patients with irritable bowel syndrome with constipation: results of two phase 3 randomized clinical trials. Am J Gastroenterol 2018;113(5):735–45.

58. Peters SL, Muir JG, Gibson PR. Review article: gut-directed hypnotherapy in the management of irritable bowel syndrome and inflammatory bowel disease. Aliment Pharmacol Ther 2015;41(11):1104–15.

59. Peters SL, Yao CK, Philpott H, et al. Randomised clinical trial: the efficacy of gut-directed hypnotherapy is similar to that of the low FODMAP diet for the treatment of irritable bowel syndrome. Aliment Pharmacol Ther 2016;44(5):447–59.

60. Chao GQ, Zhang S. Effectiveness of acupuncture to treat irritable bowel syndrome: a meta-analysis. World J Gastroenterol 2014;20:1871–7.

61. Zhao JM, Lu JH, Yin XJ, et al. Comparison of electroacupuncture and mild-warm moxibustion on brain-gut function in patients with constipation-predominant irritable bowel syndrome: a randomized controlled trial. Chin J Integr Med 2018;24(5): 328–35.

62. Lackner J, Jaccard J, Keefer L, et al. Improvement in gastrointestinal symptoms after cognitive behavior therapy for refractory irritable bowel syndrome. Gastroenterology 2018;155(1):47–57.

The Management of Chronic Pancreatitis

Vaishali Patel, MD, MHS[a], Field Willingham, MD, MPH[b],*

KEYWORDS

- Chronic • Pancreatitis • Management • Therapy • Endoscopy

KEY POINTS

- Chronic pancreatitis (CP) may remain undiagnosed for extended periods of time, until patients exhibit manifestations, such as pain and exocrine or endocrine insufficiency, or complications, such as malignancy.
- Addressing modifiable causes, monitoring to assess the response to therapy, and consultation with a multidisciplinary team are essential components in the management of CP.
- Although some patients may remain symptomatic in spite of therapy, interventions may slow progression, impact quality of life, and prevent or address complications.

INTRODUCTION

Chronic pancreatitis (CP) is the result of long-standing or recurrent inflammation of the pancreas, eventually resulting in fibrosis and loss of both islet and acinar cells. Acute pancreatitis may precede the development of CP, though there are patients who develop manifestations of chronic disease without recurrent acute episodes. Conversely, most cases of acute pancreatitis do not evolve into CP. Smoking- or alcohol-related pancreatitis has a higher likelihood of progression to chronic disease. The diagnosis can easily be missed in the early stages, which presents an obstacle for therapy and allows for progression of the disease. Although patients with CP vary in the presentation and severity of symptoms, the disease can significantly impact quality of life for many patients.

MANAGEMENT GOALS

Effective treatment of CP requires recognition of the diagnosis, addressing modifiable causes for the disease (to slow progression), and management of symptoms and

Disclosures: The authors have no personal, business, or financial conflicts of interest or any funding sources to disclose that are relevant to this article.
[a] Division of Digestive Diseases, Department of Medicine, Emory University School of Medicine, 1365 Clifton Road, Northeast, Building B, Suite 1200, Atlanta, GA 30322, USA; [b] Division of Digestive Diseases, Department of Medicine, Emory University Hospital, Children's Healthcare of Atlanta, Emory University School of Medicine, 1365 Clifton Road, Northeast, Building B, Suite 1200, Atlanta, GA 30322, USA
* Corresponding author.
E-mail address: field.willingham@emory.edu

Med Clin N Am 103 (2019) 153–162
https://doi.org/10.1016/j.mcna.2018.08.012
0025-7125/19/© 2018 Elsevier Inc. All rights reserved.

complications with a multidisciplinary team. Monitoring patients to assess the outcome of therapy and to detect potential complications is crucial. Symptom recognition is important and should lead to testing to establish the diagnosis of CP. Given that there are no therapies to reverse established CP, it is imperative to establish the diagnosis so that modifiable risk factors can be addressed earlier and further damage ameliorated. Although some patients may remain symptomatic, interventions can improve quality of life for many patients.

Recognizing the disease and confirming the diagnosis is the first step in management. A biopsy of the pancreas is not required and is not available in many centers. Findings of fibrosis and atrophy can also be seen in asymptomatic patients, elderly patients, patients who smoke, and those with renal failure or diabetes. Imaging findings or tests of pancreatic function can be used to diagnose CP, though these tests may be negative in the early stages of the disease. Missing the diagnosis during the early stages averts the opportunity to intervene and may allow progression to advanced stages. Imaging features, such as atrophy of the pancreas, dilatation of the pancreatic duct, and pancreatic calcifications, can take between 5 and 10 years to develop and are pathognomonic of CP.[1] Pancreatic calcifications may be missed on imaging with MRI/magnetic resonance cholangiopancreatography (MRCP) but are visualized well on computed tomography (CT) scans with a pancreatic contrast protocol or on radiograph (**Fig. 1**). Calcifications are more likely to be seen in patients with pancreatitis due to alcohol and or smoking and may be seen in hereditary or tropical pancreatitis. Pancreatic ductal anatomy is well visualized by MRI/MRCP (**Fig. 2**). Endoscopic ultrasonography (EUS) is highly sensitive in detecting changes of CP. The Rosemont criteria describe a scheme for interpreting major and minor imaging features (**Fig. 3**) to diagnose CP.[2] EUS has a high sensitivity but low specificity for the diagnosis of CP given that some EUS findings may be nonspecific and nondiagnostic for CP. These imaging modalities also evaluate for and may find complications of CP, such as progression to adenocarcinoma.

Indirect tests of pancreatic function, such as fecal elastase measurement, may permit the diagnosis of pancreatic exocrine insufficiency, a common complication of CP. Fecal elastase is a sensitive test for pancreatic insufficiency. However, the

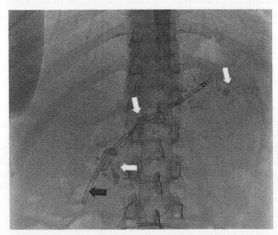

Fig. 1. Radiograph of CP during endoscopic retrograde cholangiopancreatography. Arrows indicate diffuse pancreatic calcifications (*yellow*) and transpapillary plastic pancreatic stent (*red*).

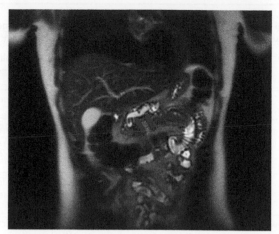

Fig. 2. MRI scan of CP (*arrows* indicate pancreatic duct dilatation).

test may also be abnormal in patients with prior small bowel surgeries or diarrhea of other causes. Direct tests of pancreatic function involve the collection of pancreatic secretions following the administration of the hormone secretin with subsequent analysis for bicarbonate concentration and secretion of various proteins. These tests are not widely performed. Direct or indirect biochemical tests may be helpful when the diagnosis is questionable or the imaging is equivocal.

The toxic-metabolic, idiopathic, genetic, autoimmune, recurrent and severe acute pancreatitis obstructive classification system[2] describes common causes for CP (**Table 1**). Confirmation of the underlying cause of CP permits therapy aimed at the source and lifestyle modification. Pancreatitis does not develop in all patients who drink alcohol; however, long-term exposure to large amounts (5 or more drinks per day) is a risk factor for CP. Smoking is also a known risk factor for CP. Patients with CP who continue to smoke or drink alcohol are at risk for worsening of their disease, including formation of calcifications as well as intraductal adenocarcinoma. Alcohol and tobacco cessation are of critical importance.

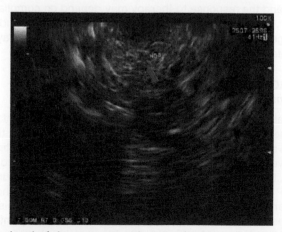

Fig. 3. EUS of the head of the pancreas with major features of CP including hyperechoic strands and lobularity (*arrow* indicates head of pancreas).

Table 1
Causes associated with chronic pancreatitis: toxic-metabolic, idiopathic, genetic, autoimmune, recurrent and severe acute pancreatitis obstructive classification system

Toxic-Metabolic	Alcoholic, tobacco smoking, hypercalcemia (hyperparathyroidism), hyperlipidemia (rare and controversial), chronic renal failure, medications, toxins
Idiopathic	Early onset, late onset, tropical (tropical calcific pancreatitis, fibro-calculous pancreatic diabetes), other
Genetic	Autosomal dominant (cationic trypsinogen codon 29 and 122 mutations), autosomal recessive/modifier genes (CFTR mutations, SPINK1 mutations, cationic trypsinogen codon 16, 22, 23 mutations, alpha-1 antitrypsin deficiency)
Autoimmune	Isolated autoimmune chronic pancreatitis, syndromic autoimmune CP (Sjogren syndrome, inflammatory bowel disease, primary biliary cirrhosis)
Recurrent and Severe Acute Pancreatitis	Postnecrotic (severe acute pancreatitis), recurrent acute pancreatitis, vascular diseases/ischemia, postirradiation
Obstructive	Pancreatic divisum, sphincter of Oddi disorders (controversial), duct obstruction (such as tumor), preampullary duodenal wall cysts, posttraumatic pancreatic duct scars

Abbreviations: CTFR, cystic fibrosis transmembrane conductance regulator; SPINK 1, serine protease inhibitor Kazal type-1.
From Conwell DL, Lee LS, Yadav D, et al. American Pancreatic Association Practice Guidelines in Chronic Pancreatitis: Evidence-Based Report on Diagnostic Guidelines. Pancreas 2014;43(8):1143–62; with permission.

Management of symptoms is key in impacting quality of life in patients with CP. The main symptom experienced by patients with CP is chronic abdominal pain, often postprandial in nature. Daily, continuous pain is associated with a reduced quality of life. It spurs patients to seek medical care and make emergency department visits and is responsible for a large percentage of health care utilization and CP-related medical costs.[3] A subset of patients who progress to substantial tissue destruction may eventually develop exocrine or endocrine insufficiency. This complication may occur over years. Symptoms of exocrine insufficiency may include fatty diarrhea, malabsorption, and weight loss, whereas endocrine insufficiency leads to diabetes. These symptoms vary in severity, and the response to therapy may depend on compliance with medication and dietary recommendations and abstinence from alcohol and tobacco exposure. The management of CP can be challenging, and patients may have ongoing symptoms in spite of maximal therapy.

PHARMACOLOGIC AND MEDICAL STRATEGIES
Pain Management

Pain has the greatest impact on quality of life and disability for patients with CP. In order to assess the response to therapy, it is beneficial to establish the severity and character of pain as well as the reduction in quality of life before initiating therapy. Previous studies have shown a 33% to 50% pain relief rate with only medical therapy.[1] In patients with CP, the mechanism of pain is complex. Emerging literature suggests that patients with CP have larger nociceptive neurons with surrounding inflammation. These neurons are stimulated by trypsin, a pancreatic enzyme. This stimulation increases the sensation of pain, in addition to pain caused by inflammation and ischemia. Furthermore, hyperalgesia is caused by sensitization of secondary spinal cord neurons that communicate with the nociceptive neurons. This circuit also leads to allodynia. Lastly, connections between the second-order neurons and third-order neurons in the brain that transmit to the limbic system and somatosensory cortex create the sensation of pain and also evoke the emotion of suffering. Notably, the placebo response in these patients is estimated to be at least 20%. As in other patients with chronic pain, those with CP have alterations in brain microstructure and function that lead to changes in cortical organization and brain-evoked potentials.[4] Therefore, neuromodulating agents, such as gabapentoids, and selective serotonin reuptake inhibitors (SSRIs) may be effective in reducing pain in patients with CP.[5]

It is estimated by cohort and cross-sectional studies that approximately half of patients with CP are treated with opioids. Opioids should be avoided if possible. Long-term use often paradoxically increases the perception of pain as tolerance develops. The use of analgesics may be required. In this setting, it is recommended to begin with lower doses and less potent agents, such as tramadol (200–400 mg per day). Although higher doses or stronger opioids may be necessary in some cases, changes and increases should be made slowly with continued reassessment of the response to therapy. The goal should be reduction of pain and not elimination of pain. Patients with a history of addictive behavior, such as alcohol abuse or smoking, are at the highest risk of addiction to opioids. The risk of addiction specifically in patients with CP is unknown. To help reduce the use of narcotics, SSRIs, serotonin-norepinephrine reuptake inhibitors, tricyclic antidepressants, and gabapentoids can be used to work synergistically for pain control. In a randomized controlled trial of patients with CP, pregabalin 300 mg twice daily reduced pain compared with placebo and allowed for reduction of opioid use.[5] Providers should also monitor patients for signs of addictive behavior and reassess the need to initiate adjunctive medications or therapies.

Other nonanalgesic medications may be helpful for pain control in patients with CP. Small randomized studies evaluating the use of pancreatic enzymes for pain control have mixed results. The studies used varying dosages and evaluated different outcomes. Consequently, there is no standard recommendation for pancreatic enzymes for pain control; however, given the lack of significant side effects, it is often considered in patients with chronic symptoms. Octreotide has had mixed results in 4 randomized studies, is expensive and injection based, and is not considered standard therapy. Antioxidants have been evaluated in 2 large randomized trials, in which they seemed to demonstrate efficacy for pain relief in the trial with younger patients with idiopathic pancreatitis; however, they were not beneficial in a trial with older patients with alcohol- or tobacco-related pancreatitis.[6–8] Although antioxidant supplements are not in standard use, encouraging consumption of fruits and vegetables that are high in antioxidants may be a reasonable recommendation.

Exocrine Insufficiency Management

Exocrine insufficiency may manifest with steatorrhea or diarrhea, weight loss, or with other signs of malabsorption and malnutrition, such as vitamin and mineral deficiency or loss of bone health. Most commonly, exocrine insufficiency develops in patients who have had CP for more than 5 to 10 years. This insufficiency is diagnosed by a low fecal elastase level less than 200 µg/g of stool or low serum trypsin less than 20 ng/mL. A 72-hour fecal fat measurement can be used to diagnose steatorrhea; however, it is rarely performed given the inconvenience and inaccuracies associated with stool collection and analysis. Pancreatic enzyme replacement can treat exocrine insufficiency. An evaluation of the baseline nutritional status should be performed before enzyme replacement initiation. Baseline laboratory tests should include complete blood counts, a comprehensive metabolic panel, international normalized ratio, albumin and prealbumin levels, carotene, and vitamin D level. Bone mineral density testing should be considered at appropriate intervals. Approximately 90,000 United States Pharmacopeia (USP) units of lipase (10% of what the pancreas produces for each meal) is required to avoid fat malabsorption with each meal. Enteric-coated and uncoated formulations are available in the United States. A proton-pump inhibitor or H2-blocker is recommended to protect the pH-sensitive delivery capsules from the acidic environment of the stomach to allow breakdown and release in the duodenum for maximal effect where absorption is taking place. This recommendation is especially important for the nonenteric coated formulation. The dose should be taken with every meal and snack, splitting the dose during and after the meal. The dose can be increased in a weight-based manner from 50,000 USP to 90,000 USP per meal depending on the response of symptoms, such as ongoing diarrhea. For ongoing symptoms, it is recommended to check that patients are taking it correctly and taking the appropriate dose. For refractory symptoms, other causes should be considered, such as small bowel bacterial overgrowth or infectious diarrhea.

Endocrine Insufficiency Management

Endocrine insufficiency may also develop over time in patients with CP. Patients with CP may also have type 2 diabetes mellitus due to other comorbidities, such as obesity. Some patients with type I diabetes mellitus develop CP. Type 3 diabetes mellitus develops in patients with long-standing CP or patients who have significant pancreatic resection. These patients have low insulin and low glucagon levels, along with reduction in other regulatory hormones produced by islet cells, and may be more prone to treatment-induced hypoglycemia or ketoacidosis. Diabetes in this setting may increase the risk of pancreatic cancer as well, though the mechanism in this setting is unknown. This risk may be abated by hyperglycemia control with metformin.[9] It is reasonable to screen annually for diabetes with fasting plasma glucose and hemoglobin A1c levels in patients with CP and to refer to an endocrinologist for treatment if appropriate.

NONPHARMACOLOGIC STRATEGIES

Nonpharmacologic options for patients with symptoms refractory to medical therapy include endoscopic therapy, surgical management, and/or nerve block. Historically, stones or strictures causing pancreatic duct obstruction were considered one of the possible causes of pain in CP. This cause may not be the case for patients with early disease who have pain without evidence of duct obstruction. Not all patients with duct obstruction have symptoms of pain; furthermore, the degree of duct dilatation and the presence of stones may not correlate with symptoms. Endoscopic retrograde cholangiopancreatography (ERCP) with stone extraction, lithotripsy, and stricture dilation, with or without transpapillary stent placement, or surgical ductal drainage are 2 potential therapies to treat pain in CP.

Endoscopic Therapy

Patients selected for endoscopic therapy often have a dilatated main pancreatic duct (more than 5–6 mm) with an obstructing stone and/or stricture. Brushing for cytology to rule out malignancy may be considered for new strictures. Challenges to endoscopic therapy include large, impacted, or multiple stones, which may require extracorporeal shock wave lithotripsy (ESWL) or intraductal lithotripsy. Lithotripsy is an adjunctive therapy to ERCP. A previous randomized controlled trial showed that ESWL alone is equivalent to ESWL followed by ERCP for the removal of pancreatic stones and is also cost saving.[10] Various endoscopic dilators exist for the management of very severe strictures that cannot be traversed. Stones and strictures that are further from the ampulla may be less amenable to endoscopic therapy. Because the degree of duct dilatation does not correlate with symptoms, it may be difficult to correlate the degree of duct decompression following therapy with symptom relief or resolution. However, large retrospective studies evaluating the effectiveness of endoscopic therapy (including ESWL) in CP demonstrate high (approximately 80%) technical success rates and clinical success with relief of pain in 50% to 70% of carefully selected patients with amenable ductal anatomy.[11,12] Endoscopic duct decompression remains a mainstay of therapy before consideration of surgery, with ERCP, ESWL for large stones (>5 mm) before ERCP or ESWL alone (without ERCP) for small stones (<5 mm).[13]

Pain control can also be achieved endoscopically with EUS-guided neurolysis or nerve block. This pain control is achieved by injection of bupivacaine and corticosteroids in the area of the celiac plexus under EUS guidance. About 50% of patients with CP will experience reduction of pain within a few weeks following EUS-guided neurolysis, and pain relief may be short-term.[1] Patients with pain due to pancreatic cancer who have not become sensitized to pain generally may experience more effective pain relief by this method. Given this, it is not routinely recommended for patients with CP, though it is thought to be safer and more effective than CT-guided nerve block. Neurolysis with injection of absolute alcohol and thoracoscopic splanchnicectomy is not the first-line therapy but may be considered in some situations for patients with painful CP.

Surgical Therapy

Surgery is often reserved for patients who are refractory to both medical and endoscopic therapy. Surgery may be a suitable option for treatment of pain and also for complications, such as biliary or bowel obstruction. Most commonly, patients will undergo a lateral pancreaticojejunostomy or modified Puestow procedure. Dilatation of the pancreatic duct of at least 6 mm is typically required for this surgery. The surgery involves creating a longitudinal incision of the duct and anterior pancreas, stone extraction, and creation of an anastomosis with a small bowel roux limb along the longitudinal length of the pancreas. This surgery results in pain relief for 80% of patients, with 50% maintaining pain relief at 5 or more years postoperatively. A pancreaticoduodenectomy (Whipple procedure) or a duodenum-preserving pancreatic head resection (DPPHR) allows for pancreatic duct drainage along with resection of the pancreatic head, which may be required in the setting of biliary or duodenal obstruction due to an inflammatory or fibrotic mass at the head of the pancreas. The 3 forms of the DPPHR are the Frey (coring out of the pancreatic head without division of the neck, followed by longitudinal pancreaticojejunostomy), Beger (pancreatic head resection with division of the neck, preservation of the duodenum and bile duct, with pancreaticojejunostomy), and Berne (partial pancreatic head resection of the anterior capsule only with side-to-side pancreaticojejunostomy) procedures. All of these procedures seem to be equivalent in providing short-term pain relief relative to the Puestow operation but may have better long-term pain relief. However, DPPHR patients may develop exocrine and endocrine insufficiency due to resection of part of the pancreas; patients with Whipple disease may have postoperative diabetes and lower quality of life.[1] Distal pancreatectomy may be an option for patients with disease limited to the tail of the pancreas, but it is infrequently performed. Total pancreatectomy is also rarely used given the resultant profound endocrine and exocrine insufficiency. It can be paired with islet autotransplantation (TPIAT), in which the islets are collected from the resected pancreas and infused into the portal vein. They then implant into the liver, potentially reducing the severity of endocrine insufficiency and diabetes after the surgery. These procedures were previously considered in patients who had failed other interventions but are now being considered for patients with severe CP who have not had previous surgeries. It was previously estimated that pain relief occurs only in 66% of patients who undergo total pancreatectomy, and 55% of patients will be insulin dependent after surgery. More recent studies report pain relief rates of 72% to 86%, with 47% to 55% morbidity and 1.4% to 6.0% mortality.[14] Patients without insulin dependence after surgery may develop endocrine insufficiency. The risk of diabetes is inversely correlated with islet cell yield (which is lower in patients who have undergone previous surgical interventions, such as the Puestow procedure). TPAIT is primarily considered in patients with pain and debilitating CP who have not responded to medical, endoscopic, and/or surgical therapies. The impairment in patients' quality of life should be significant enough to outweigh the risk of insulin dependence and the requirement for lifelong pancreatic enzyme replacement therapy.

Pain relief was found to be equivalent between patients undergoing endoscopic therapy (sphincterotomy, stricture dilation, stone extraction, and stenting) or surgery (drainage, DPPHR, or Whipple) at 1 year following intervention in one study of 72 patients.[15] However, a second study with 39 patients was stopped early because of a significant benefit in the surgery group of either partial or complete pain relief at 24 months and at 5 years,[16,17] with equivalent pancreatic function, quality of life, and costs in subsequent analyses.

EVALUATION, ADJUSTMENT, AND RECURRENCE

For patients with pain, reevaluation of symptoms, and the response to therapy should be performed at each visit, with adjustments to doses of analgesics as needed. Adjunctive agents can be added as noted previously. Attempts to wean narcotic use should be made regularly. Similarly, assessment of nutritional status should be repeated at subsequent visits after initiation of pancreatic enzyme supplementation; the daily dose can be increased if needed. A referral to nutrition services may be beneficial. Counseling for tobacco and alcohol abstinence reduces recurrent episodes, reduces pain, slows the progression of disease, decreases the risk of complications and the risk of malignancy, and prolongs life.[18] If the provider is not proficient in counseling methods, referrals for substance use/abuse support should be placed, including behavioral interventions.[19] Screening for pancreatic malignancy with MRI or EUS on an annual basis is recommended for patients with hereditary causes of CP.[20] Dietary modification and healthy lifestyle choices are critical. Patients should adhere to a multiple small meal, low-fat diet. Furthermore, supplementation of vitamin D and calcium and a bone density scan should be provided to prevent osteopenia, osteoporosis, and fractures. Certain causes of pancreatitis may require specific treatment, such as steroid therapy for autoimmune pancreatitis. Other treatable complications that may be contributing to symptoms should be ruled out, such as pseudocysts, biliary obstruction, duodenal obstruction, or malignancy. These complications may be detected on cross-sectional imaging. If present, these patients can be referred for endoscopic therapy or surgery as appropriate.

SUMMARY AND FUTURE CONSIDERATIONS

The management of CP may require medical, endoscopic, and surgical modalities of treatment. A multidisciplinary approach for the management of patients with CP is often required. Primary care providers build long-term relationships and may be the first to evaluate patients before subspecialty referral. Management should focus on abstinence from exposures, such as alcohol and tobacco. Dietary recommendations include multiple small meals per day and healthy, low-fat foods. Patients should be monitored for complications. Endocrine and exocrine insufficiency may be addressed with medical therapy, pancreatic enzyme replacement therapy, and vitamin supplementation. A pain control regimen should be developed that avoids narcotic medications. Being aware of the pitfalls and challenges and recognizing potential complications of CP allow for appropriate diagnostic testing to be performed and timely referrals to be placed when indicated. Providers may also support patients with refractory symptoms with counseling, behavioral therapy, and support groups through the National Pancreas Foundation. With proper intervention, the health and quality of life for our patients with CP can be greatly improved.

REFERENCES

1. Forsmark CE. Management of chronic pancreatitis. Gastroenterology 2013; 144(6):1282–91.
2. Conwell DL, Lee LS, Yadav D, et al. American Pancreatic Association practice guidelines in chronic pancreatitis: evidence-based report on diagnostic guidelines. Pancreas 2014;43(8):1143–62.
3. Mullady DK, Yadav D, Amann ST, et al. NAPS2 consortium. Type of pain, pain-associated complications, quality of life, disability and resource utilisation in chronic pancreatitis: a prospective cohort study. Gut 2011;60:77–84.
4. Pasricha PJ. Unraveling the mystery of pain in chronic pancreatitis. Nat Rev Gastroenterol Hepatol 2012;9:140–51.
5. Olesen SS, Bouwense SA, Wilder-Smith OH, et al. Pregabalin reduces pain in patients with chronic pancreatitis in a randomized controlled trial. Gastroenterology 2011;141:536–43.
6. Siriwardena AK, Mason JM, Sheen AJ, et al. Antioxidant therapy does not reduce pain in patients with chronic pancreatitis: the ANTICIPATE study. Gastroenterology 2012;143:655–63.
7. Bhardwaj P, Garg PK, Maulik SK, et al. A randomized controlled trial of antioxidant supplementation for pain relief in patients with chronic pancreatitis. Gastroenterology 2009;136:149–59.
8. Forsmark CE, Liddle R. The challenging task of treating painful chronic pancreatitis. Gastroenterology 2012;143:533–5.
9. Cui Y, Andersen DK. Diabetes and pancreatic cancer. Endocr Relat Cancer 2012; 19:F9–26.
10. Dumonceau JM, Costamagna G, Tringali A. Treatment for painful chronic pancreatitis: extracorporeal shock wave lithotripsy versus endoscopic treatment: a randomized controlled trial. Gut 2007;5:545–52.
11. Clarke B, Slivka A, Tomizawa Y, et al. Endoscopic therapy is effective for chronic pancreatitis. Clin Gastroenterol Hepatol 2012;10:795–802.
12. Rosch T, Daniel S, Sholz M, et al. Endoscopic treatment of chronic pancreatitis: a multicenter study of 1000 patients with long-term follow-up. Endoscopy 2002;34: 765–71.
13. Dumonceau JM, Delhaye M, Tringali A. Endoscopic treatment of chronic pancreatitis: European society of gastrointestinal endoscopy (ESGE): clinical guideline. Endoscopy 2012;44:784–96.
14. Sutherland DE, Radosevich DM, Bellin MD, et al. Total pancreatectomy and islet autotransplantation for chronic pancreatitis. J Am Coll Surg 2012;214(4): 409–24.

15. Dite P, Ruzicka M, Zboril V, et al. A prospective, randomized trial comparing endoscopic and surgical therapy for chronic pancreatitis. Endoscopy 2003;35: 553–8.
16. Cahen DL, Gouma DJ, Nio Y, et al. Endoscopic versus surgical drainage of the pancreatic duct in painful chronic pancreatitis. N Engl J Med 2007;356:676–84.
17. Cahen DL, Gouma DJ, Laramee P, et al. Long-term outcomes of endoscopic vs surgical drainage of the pancreatic duct in patients with chronic pancreatitis. Gastroenterology 2011;141:1690–5.
18. Lowenfels AB, Maisonneuve P. Defining the role of smoking in chronic pancreatitis. Clin Gastroenterol Hepatol 2011;9:196–7.
19. Drewes AM, Bouwense SAW, Campbell CM, et al. Guidelines for the understanding and management of pain in chronic pancreatitis. Pancreatology 2017;17: 720–31.
20. Canto MI, Harinck F, Hruban RH, et al. International Cancer of the Pancreas Screening (CAPS) Consortium summit on the management of patients with increased risk for familial pancreatic cancer. Gut 2013;62(3):339–47.

Pancreatic Cysts
Sinister Findings or Incidentalomas?

Olaya I. Brewer Gutierrez, MD[a],
Anne Marie Lennon, MD, PhD[b,c,d,e],*

KEYWORDS

- Pancreatic cysts • Pancreatic cystic neoplasm • IPMN • Mucin producing cyst
- Mucinous cystic neoplasm • MCN

KEY POINTS

- Pancreatic cysts are common and are found in up to 13% of people aged between 70 and 80 years.
- Two types of cysts, intraductal papillary mucinous neoplasm (IPMN) and mucinous cystic neoplasm (MCN), are precancerous cysts that can develop into pancreatic cancer in a small number of cases.
- Several other types of pancreatic cysts, such as pseudocysts and serous cysts, have no malignant potential.
- Guidelines recommend surveillance of patients with an IPMN or an MCN.
- Patients with an IPMN or an MCN with concerning features should be referred to a multidisciplinary group for consideration of surgical resection.

Funding: This work was supported by the Lustgarten Foundation for Pancreatic Cancer Research, Susan Wojcicki and Dennis Troper, The Sol Goldman Center for Pancreatic Cancer Research, The Benjamin Baker Scholarship, and the National Institutes of Health Grants P50-CA62924.
[a] Division of Gastroenterology and Hepatology, Johns Hopkins Medical Institution, The Johns Hopkins Hospital, Sheikh Zayed Building, 1800 Orleans Street, Suite M2058, Baltimore, MD 21287, USA; [b] Medicine, Multidisciplinary Pancreatic Cyst Clinic, The Johns Hopkins Medical Institutions, 1800 Orleans Street, Room 7125J, Baltimore, MD 21231, USA; [c] Surgery, Multidisciplinary Pancreatic Cyst Clinic, The Johns Hopkins Medical Institutions, 1800 Orleans Street, Room 7125J, Baltimore, MD 21231, USA; [d] Oncology, Multidisciplinary Pancreatic Cyst Clinic, The Johns Hopkins Medical Institutions, 1800 Orleans Street, Room 7125J, Baltimore, MD 21231, USA; [e] Radiology, Multidisciplinary Pancreatic Cyst Clinic, The Johns Hopkins Medical Institutions, 1800 Orleans Street, Room 7125J, Baltimore, MD 21231, USA
* Corresponding author. Division of Gastroenterology and Hepatology, Johns Hopkins Medical Institution, 1800 Orleans Street, Room 7125J, Baltimore, MD 21231, USA.
E-mail address: amlennon@jhmi.edu

Med Clin N Am 103 (2019) 163–172
https://doi.org/10.1016/j.mcna.2018.08.004
0025-7125/19/© 2018 Elsevier Inc. All rights reserved.

INTRODUCTION
How Common Are Pancreatic Cysts?

Pancreatic cysts are a biologically heterogeneous group of lesions that range from completely benign to malignant.[1,2] Pancreatic cysts are incidentally identified in 2.6% of patients who undergo a computed tomography (CT) scan[3] and in 2.4% to 13.5% of individuals who have an MRI.[4,5] The prevalence increases with age. This is highlighted in a study by de Jong and colleagues[5] that analyzed 2803 sequential subjects who underwent MRI. They identified a pancreatic cyst in 0.23% of individuals aged 18 to 39 years, 1.3% of people aged 40 to 49 years, 2.6% of individuals aged 50 to 59 years, 3.6% of people 60 to 69 years, and 10.6% of individuals aged 70 to 79 years.[5]

Why the Interest in Pancreatic Cysts?

Pancreatic adenocarcinoma has a 5-year survival rate of only 8%[6] and is predicted to become the second most common cause of death due to cancer by 2030.[7] There are 3 precursors to pancreatic adenocarcinoma: pancreatic intraepithelial neoplasia (PanIN), intraductal papillary mucinous neoplasm (IPMN), and mucinous cystic neoplasm (MCN).[8] PanINs lesions are small lesions that currently cannot be seen except with a microscope following surgical resection. In contrast, IPMNs and MCNs are pancreatic cysts, and are easily identified with CT or MRI. The identification of IPMNs and MCNs offers the possibility of earlier detection of pancreatic adenocarcinoma.[8]

Which Imaging Tests Should Be Used to Assess Pancreatic Cysts?

In general, magnetic resonance cholangiopancreatography (MRCP) is considered the imaging test of choice for the surveillance of a pancreatic cyst.[1] MRCP is more accurate than CT for evaluating communication between the pancreatic cyst and the main pancreatic duct (MPD), which is a key feature for identifying IPMNs. It has the additional benefit of having no radiation exposure. However, nether MRI nor CT is perfect at differentiating IPMNs and MCNs from other types of cysts. A systematic review by Jones and colleagues[9] found that CT and MRI had an accuracy of between 39% to 84%, and 50% to 88%, respectively, for identifying the type of cyst. Endoscopic ultrasound (EUS) may be considered if the diagnosis is unclear and when the results are likely to alter management.[1] It is the best test for identifying mural nodules, with a sensitivity of 75%, compared with 47% for CT, and similar specificity.[10] In addition, EUS with fine-needle aspiration (EUS-FNA) can be performed and cyst fluid and cells evaluated. The most commonly used test is cyst fluid carcinoembryonic antigen (CEA). Using a cutoff of higher than 192 ng/mL, it has a sensitivity of 63%, and specificity of 93% for differentiating an IPMN or MCN from other types of cysts.[11] A low (<250 IU/L) cyst fluid amylase level can exclude a pseudocyst with 98% specificity; however, high amylase levels seen in multiple types of cysts is not useful.[12] The presence of mucin on cytology is suggestive of an IPMN or MCN. Cytology is also useful for evaluating for the presence of high-grade dysplasia or cancer within the cyst. However, although the specificity of cytology is greater than 90%, it is limited by its sensitivity of just greater than 50%.[11]

Types and Management of Pancreatic Cysts

Pancreatic cysts can be classified as benign, premalignant, and malignant (**Table 1**). Understanding this classification is crucial because patient management is based on the risk of malignant transformation.

Table 1
Types of pancreatic cysts

Cyst Type	Sex	Age	Pancreatic Localization	Morphology	Communication with MPD	Malignancy Risk
Benign						
Pseudocyst	♂ or ♀	…	Entire pancreas	Unilocular or single chamber	+ or –	–
SCA	♀	60	Entire pancreas	Microcystic or tiny cysts	–	–
Malignant Potential						
IPMN	♂ or ♀	65	Head	Unilocular, septated, + + or – dilated MPD	+++	+++
MCN	♀	40	Body or tail	Unilocular	–	+++
Malignant						
SPN	♀	30	Body or tail	Mixed solid and cystic	–	+
PanNET	♂ or ♀	50	Entire pancreas	Associated mass	–	+

♀, female gender; ♂, male gender.
Abbreviations: PanNET, pancreatic neuroendocrine tumor; SPN, solid-pseudopapillary neoplasia.

Benign Cysts

Pancreatic pseudocyst

Pseudocysts almost always occur in patients with known history of acute and chronic pancreatitis. It is important to remember that acute pancreatitis can be caused by an undiagnosed pancreatic cancer. EUS should be performed in individuals with acute pancreatitis aged older than 40 years with acute pancreatitis and no cause because of the risk of pancreatic cancer causing acute pancreatitis in this age group.[1] Key features on the history are the presence of acute onset of epigastric pain, nausea, and/or vomiting; the presence of gallstones; or a history of significant alcohol consumption or high triglyceride levels. On imaging, pseudocysts are well-defined and found either within or adjacent to the pancreas; they can be single or multiple. Initially, the wall is thin but may thicken as the pseudocyst matures.[13] The cyst may contain debris or necrosis. In cases in which the diagnosis is unclear, EUS-FNA with cyst fluid analysis can be helpful. Key characteristics of the fluid are: brownish color, high amylase levels (>250 U/L), and low CEA levels (<5 ng/mL).[14] Pseudocysts are benign and do not require surveillance[1] (**Table 2**).

Serous cystadenoma

Serous cystadenomas (SCAs) represent 16% of all resected pancreatic cystic neoplasias.[15] Approximately two-thirds occur in women. They can be located anywhere within the pancreas and are typically single cysts. The risk of malignant transformation is exceedingly small. A large systematic review of more than 2500 subjects with SCAs found a 0.1% risk cancer developing within a SCA.[16] SCAs are usually asymptomatic and rarely cause abdominal pain, pancreatitis, or jaundice. The most common appearance on imaging is a microcystic cyst in which the cyst is made up of multiple tiny cysts that have a honeycomb appearance (**Fig. 1**A). A central scar with calcification is pathognomonic but is only present in 15% to 30% of cases. If the diagnosis is unclear, EUS-FNA can be performed. The cyst fluid analysis typically shows a low CEA (<5 ng/mL).[17] Molecular analysis of cyst fluid will show a mutation in the *VHL* gene with no mutations in *GNAS* or *KRAS*.[18] SCAs are benign and surveillance is not required[1] (see **Table 2**).

Cysts with Malignant Potential

Mucinous cystic neoplasms

MCNs represent 24% of all resected pancreatic cysts.[15] They are usually single cysts, typically present in women aged between 40 and 60 years, and are located in the body or tail of the pancreas in greater than 90% of cases.[19] On imaging, an MCN is a single cyst, with or without division or septa, that does not connect or communicate with the MPD (**Fig. 1**B). The cyst fluid typically has a high CEA level of greater than 192 ng/mL, and mucin may be seen on cytology.[12] The presence of a *KRAS* mutation in the cyst fluid is further evidence supporting the diagnosis of an MCN.

Intraductal papillary mucinous neoplasms

IPMNs are the most common type of pancreatic cyst, making up 38% of all resected pancreatic cysts.[15] They are equally common in men and women, and typically present in individuals in their sixtieth and seventieth decades. They can be located anywhere within the pancreas, with 40% of subjects having multiple cysts. IPMNs are classified into 1 of 3 types, depending on whether there is involvement of the MPD. Main duct IPMNs (MD-IPMNs) have an enlarged (>5 mm) MPD (**Fig. 1**C). Branch duct IPMNs (BD-IPMN) have a normal size MPD but 1 or more cysts and can be communicating with the MPD (**Fig. 1**D). Patients who have both an enlarged MPD and 1 or more cysts are classified as having a mixed type IPMN. Determining which

Table 2
Management of pancreatic cysts

Cyst Type	Management of Asymptomatic Cysts
Benign	
Pseudocyst	No surveillance[1]
SCA	No surveillance[1]
Malignant Potential	
IPMN or MCN	Refer to a multidisciplinary group for consideration of surgical resection if there are any of the features present shown in **Table 3**[1] Asymptomatic patients with branch duct IPMNs should undergo surveillance. The interval is based on the size of the largest cyst with cysts measuring <1 cm followed every 2 y, those measuring 1–2 cm followed every year, cysts measuring 2–3 cm followed every 6 mo. The surveillance interval can be increased if the cysts are stable with no concerning features[1]
Malignant	
SPN	Surgical resection[27]
PanNET	Surgical resection if functional, or size >2 cm[27]

type of IPMN the patient has is critical because MD-IPMNs and mixed type IPMNs have a much higher risk of malignant transformation compared with BD-IPMNs (see later discussion).[20] Mucin can sometimes be seen extruding from the MPD and out of the ampulla of Vater, and is considered pathognomonic for an IPMN. Cytologic evaluation of the cyst fluid may show mucin, and may show high-grade dysplasia or

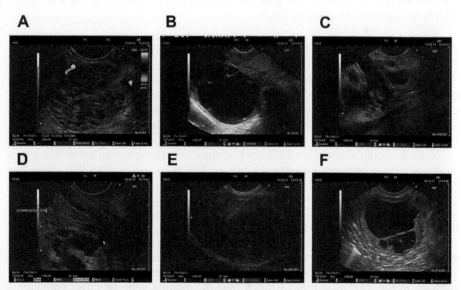

Fig. 1. Types of pancreatic cysts. (*A*) SCA. Well-defined cyst with the microcystic pattern or tiny cysts. (*B*) MCN. Single cyst with divisions or septa. (*C*) IPMN, main duct type. Dilation of the main pancreatic duct greater than 5 mm with a solid component or lump within the duct. (*D*) IPMN, branch duct type. Cyst with septa and communication with the MPD. (*E*) Solid-pseudopapillary neoplasm. Cystic and solid mass, well-defined. (*F*) Cystic pancreatic neuroendocrine tumors. Well-defined cyst with a thickened wall and septa. (*Courtesy of* A.M. Lennon MD, PhD, Baltimore, MD.)

adenocarcinoma.[11] Other helpful tests are the cyst fluid CEA levels, which are typically elevated (>192 ng/mL).[12] The presence of a *KRAS* mutation can be seen in either an IPMN or an MCN, whereas a *GNAS* mutations occur almost exclusively in IPMNs.[18]

The Risk of Intraductal Papillary Mucinous Neoplasms and Mucinous Cystic Neoplasms Developing into Pancreatic Cancer

One of the key questions is: what is the risk of an IPMN or MCN developing into pancreatic adenocarcinoma? In modern studies based on subjects who underwent surgical resection, the risk of an MCN harboring an invasive cancer varies between 4%[19] to 12%.[21] A recent systematic review and meta-analysis, found that, in the absence of symptoms or concerning features, the risk of an MCN that measured less than 4 cm harboring an invasive cancer was 0.03%.[22]

In IPMNs, MD-IPMN and mixed type IPMNs have a much higher risk of malignant transformation compared with BD-IPMNs, with 62% (range 36%–100%) of patients who undergo surgical resection found to have high-grade dysplasia or invasive cancer.[20] The risk of malignant transformation in BD-IPMNs is less clear. One group, using SEER data (Surveillance, Epidemiology and End Results program), estimated the lifetime risk to be 2.8% (95% CI 1.8%–4.0%).[23] A more recent systematic review and meta-analysis evaluated 3236 subjects with IPMNs, and divided them into those with concerning features (a mural nodule or a dilated MPD) or no concerning features. The pooled cumulative incidence of high-grade dysplasia or pancreatic adenocarcinoma in the group with concerning features was 1.95% at 1 year, 9.77% at 5 years, and 25% at 10 years, versus 0.02% at 1 year, 3.12% at 5 years, and 7.77% at 10 years in the group with no concerning features.[24] Two prospective, multicenter studies that will provide greater clarity of the true risk of malignant transformation of IPMNs and MCNs are currently enrolling subjects.

Management of Intraductal Papillary Mucinous Neoplasms and Mucinous Cystic Neoplasms

The first decision is whether surveillance is appropriate. Patients who would not consider surgical resection, or have comorbidities that would preclude surgical resection, should not undergo surveillance of their cysts.[1] The second question is whether there are any features that are associated with the presence of high-grade dysplasia or invasive cancer. The presence of any of the features highlighted in **Table 3** should warrant an EUS and referral to large-volume center that has a multidisciplinary team for further evaluation.[1] This is based on data that show that the mortality for pancreatic surgery is significantly lower at high-volume centers (3.3% in centers that perform more than 20 pancreaticoduodenectomies per year vs 14.7% in centers performing fewer than 5 pancreaticoduodenectomies per year).[25] A review by a multidisciplinary group has been shown to alter the management of 30% of patients seen, including decreasing the number of patients referred for surgical resection by 50%.[26] Patients with IPMNs and MCNs without these features should undergo surveillance as outlined in **Table 2**. Patients whose cyst increases in the size by 4 mm or more over 12 months with no other concerning features should have a shorter interval MRI or EUS[1] (see **Table 3**). Patients who develop concerning features (see **Table 3**) should be referred to a multidisciplinary group for further evaluation. Almost all expert groups recommend long-term surveillance of patients with IPMNs and MCNs.[1,20,27] For patients older than 75 years, the decision of continuing surveillance should be individualized based on life expectancy, comorbidities, and discussion with the patient.[1]

Table 3
Management of intraductal papillary mucinous neoplasms and mucinous cystic neoplasms with concerning features

Management	Concerning Features		
	Symptoms or Laboratory Finding	Imaging Finding	Other
Refer to multidisciplinary group for further evaluation and consideration of surgical resection	• Jaundice[a] • Acute pancreatitis[a] • Elevated CA 19–9	• Mural nodule or solid component[b] • Dilation of the MPD >5 mm • Focal dilation of the MPD[c] • Obstructive lesion • IPMN or MCN ≥ 3 cm	• HGD or cancer on cytology
Perform short interval MRI or EUS[d]	• New onset or worsening DM	• Rapid increase in cyst size (>3 mm/y)[e]	—

Abbreviations: CA, cancer antigen; DM, diabetes mellitus; HGD, high-grade dysplasia.
[a] Secondary to cyst.
[b] Either within the cyst or in the pancreatic parenchyma.
[c] Concerning for MD-IPMN.
[d] Conditional recommendation; very low quality of evidence.
[e] During surveillance.
Modified from Elta GH, Enestvedt BK, Sauer B, et al. ACG clinical guideline: diagnosis and management of pancreatic cysts. Am J Gastroenterol 2018;113(4):468; with permission.

Malignant cysts

Solid-pseudopapillary neoplasms Solid-pseudopapillary neoplasms are a rare type of cyst that typically present in women in their twentieth decade. They are single cysts with a cystic and solid appearance that can be located anywhere within the pancreas[28] (**Fig. 1E**). The diagnosis can usually be made on CT or MRI. Cytology obtained following EUS-FNA is highly sensitive and can be used in cases in which the diagnosis is unclear.[29] They are associated with a risk of metastases in 8% and surgical resection is recommended[1,27,28] (see **Table 2**).

Cystic pancreatic neuroendocrine tumors Cystic degeneration of a pancreatic neuroendocrine tumor (PanNET) can occur. These can be associated with the genetic syndrome multiple endocrine neoplasia type 1, which involves germline mutation of the MEN1 tumor suppressor gene and predisposes to endocrine tumors of the pituitary, parathyroid, and pancreas. On imaging, they are often single cysts with a thick, hyperenhancing wall cyst on CT during the arterial phase (**Fig. 1F**). EUS-FNA is able to confirm the diagnosis in 73% to 78% of cases.[30] Cyst fluid analysis will show a low CEA (<5 ng/mL). Functional PanNET should undergo surgical resection, as well as those measuring 2 cm or more. There is significant debate about whether a PanNET between 1 and 2 cm requires surgical resection, and these patients should be referred to a multidisciplinary group for review (see **Table 2**).

Surveillance after surgery

Patients with IPMNs who undergo surgical resection require life-long surveillance of the remnant pancreas because IPMNs can recur, and pancreatic cancer can develop in the remnant.[31] Patients with malignant cysts, such as pancreatic adenocarcinoma or neuroendocrine tumor, are followed per standard cancer surveillance protocols for 5 years. Pseudocysts, serous cysts, and MCNs without invasive cancer do not require any surveillance following resection.

FUTURE CONSIDERATIONS

CT, MRI, EUS, cyst fluid CEA, and cytology are imperfect at determining the cyst type and the presence of high-grade dysplasia. New promising technology includes mini-microscope probes, called needle confocal laser endomicroscopy, which can be placed through an EUS-FNA needle into the cyst and provide real-time imaging of the cyst wall.[32-34] New mini-biopsy forceps that can be passed through an EUS-FNA needle have been developed and initial studies seem promising.[35,36] Whole exome sequencing has been performed of IPMNs, MCNs, SCAs, and solid-pseudopapillary neoplasms.[37] This has shown that different types of cysts have specific genetic profiles associated with them. SCAs are associated with mutations in the *VHL*, MCNs have a *KRAS* mutation, whereas IPMNs will have *KRAS* or *GNAS* mutation in greater than 90% of cases.[18] The use of EUS-FNA with molecular marker analysis identified 30% of cysts that were benign and did not require surveillance.[38] Several groups have published early molecular marker studies that show promise for identifying IPMNs with high-grade dysplasia or early cancer; however, further studies are required to validate these preliminary results.[39-41]

REFERENCES

1. Elta GH, Enestvedt BK, Sauer BG, et al. ACG clinical guideline: diagnosis and management of pancreatic cysts. Am J Gastroenterol 2018;113(4):464–79.
2. Vege SS, Ziring B, Jain R, et al. American Gastroenterological Association institute guideline on the diagnosis and management of asymptomatic neoplastic pancreatic cysts. Gastroenterology 2015;148:819–22.
3. Laffan TA, Horton KM, Klein AP, et al. Prevalence of unsuspected pancreatic cysts on MDCT. AJR Am J Roentgenol 2008;191:802–7.
4. Lee KS, Sekhar A, Rofsky NM, et al. Prevalence of incidental pancreatic cysts in the adult population on MR imaging. Am J Gastroenterol 2010;105:2079–84.
5. de Jong K, Nio CY, Hermans JJ, et al. High prevalence of pancreatic cysts detected by screening magnetic resonance imaging examinations. Clin Gastroenterol Hepatol 2010;8:806–11.
6. Howlander N, et al. SEER Cancer Statistics Review. 1975-2011. 2014. Available at: http://seer.cancer.gov/csr/1975_2011/.
7. Rahib L, Smith BD, Aizenberg R, et al. Projecting cancer incidence and deaths to 2030: the unexpected burden of thyroid, liver, and pancreas cancers in the United States. Cancer Res 2014;74:2913–21.
8. Lennon AM, Wolfgang CL, Canto MI, et al. The early detection of pancreatic cancer: what will it take to diagnose and treat curable pancreatic neoplasia? Cancer Res 2014;74:3381–9.
9. Jones MJ, Buchanan AS, Neal CP, et al. Imaging of indeterminate pancreatic cystic lesions: a systematic review. Pancreatology 2013;13:436–42.
10. Zhong N, Zhang L, Takahashi N, et al. Histologic and imaging features of mural nodules in mucinous pancreatic cysts. Clin Gastroenterol Hepatol 2012;10:192–8, 198 e1-2.
11. Thornton GD, McPhail MJ, Nayagam S, et al. Endoscopic ultrasound guided fine needle aspiration for the diagnosis of pancreatic cystic neoplasms: a meta-analysis. Pancreatology 2013;13:48–57.
12. Ngamruengphong S, Lennon AM. Analysis of Pancreatic Cyst Fluid. Surg Pathol Clin 2016;9:677–84.
13. Lennon AM, Maguchi H. Evaluation of cystic lesions by EUS, MRI and CT. In: Beger HG, Buchler MW, Kozarek R, et al, editors. The pancreas – an integrated

textbook of basic science medicine and surgery. Cambridge (England): Wiley-Blackwell; 2018.

14. Ngamruengphong S, Bartel MJ, Raimondo M. Cyst carcinoembryonic antigen in differentiating pancreatic cysts: a meta-analysis. Dig Liver Dis 2013;45:920–6.

15. Valsangkar NP, Morales-Oyarvide V, Thayer SP, et al. 851 resected cystic tumors of the pancreas: a 33-year experience at the Massachusetts General Hospital. Surgery 2012;152:S4–12.

16. Jais B, Rebours V, Malleo G, et al. Serous cystic neoplasm of the pancreas: a multinational study of 2622 patients under the auspices of the International Association of Pancreatology and European Pancreatic Club (European Study Group on Cystic Tumors of the Pancreas). Gut 2016;65:305–12.

17. van der Waaij LA, van Dullemen HM, Porte RJ. Cyst fluid analysis in the differential diagnosis of pancreatic cystic lesions: a pooled analysis. Gastrointest Endosc 2005;62:383–9.

18. Springer S, Wang Y, Dal Molin M, et al. A combination of molecular markers and clinical features improve the classification of pancreatic cysts. Gastroenterology 2015;149:1501–10.

19. Yamao K, Yanagisawa A, Takahashi K, et al. Clinicopathological features and prognosis of mucinous cystic neoplasm with ovarian-type stroma: a multi-institutional study of the Japan pancreas society. Pancreas 2011;40:67–71.

20. Tanaka M, Fernández-Del Castillo C. Revisions of international consensus Fukuoka guidelines for the management of IPMN of the pancreas. Pancreatology 2017;17:738–53.

21. Crippa S, Salvia R, Warshaw AL, et al. Mucinous cystic neoplasm of the pancreas is not an aggressive entity: lessons from 163 resected patients. Ann Surg 2008; 247:571–9.

22. Nilsson LN, Keane MG, Shamali A, et al. Nature and management of pancreatic mucinous cystic neoplasm (MCN): a systematic review of the literature. Pancreatology 2016;16:1028–36.

23. Scheiman JM, Hwang JH, Moayyedi P. American gastroenterological association technical review on the diagnosis and management of asymptomatic neoplastic pancreatic cysts. Gastroenterology 2015;148:824–48.e22.

24. Choi SH, Park SH, Kim KW, et al. Progression of unresected intraductal papillary mucinous neoplasms of the pancreas to cancer: a systematic review and meta-analysis. Clin Gastroenterol Hepatol 2017;15:1509–20.e4.

25. de Wilde RF, Besselink MG, van der Tweel I, et al. Impact of nationwide centralization of pancreaticoduodenectomy on hospital mortality. Br J Surg 2012;99: 404–10.

26. Lennon AM, Manos LL, Hruban RH, et al. Role of a multidisciplinary clinic in the management of patients with pancreatic cysts: a single-center cohort study. Ann Surg Oncol 2014;21(11):3668–74.

27. European Study Group on Cystic Tumours of the Pancreas. European evidence-based guidelines on pancreatic cystic neoplasms. Gut 2018;67:789–804.

28. Law JK, Ahmed A, Singh VK, et al. A systematic review of solid-pseudopapillary neoplasms: are these rare lesions? Pancreas 2014;43:331–7.

29. Law JK, Stoita A, Wever W, et al. Endoscopic ultrasound-guided fine needle aspiration improves the pre-operative diagnostic yield of solid-pseudopapillary neoplasm of the pancreas: an international multicenter case series (with video). Surg Endosc 2014;28:2592–8.

30. Kim TS, Fernandez-del Castillo C. Diagnosis and management of pancreatic cystic neoplasms. Hematol Oncol Clin North Am 2015 Aug;29(4):655–74.

31. He J, Cameron JL, Ahuja N, et al. Is it necessary to follow patients after resection of a benign pancreatic intraductal papillary mucinous neoplasm? J Am Coll Surg 2013;216:657–65 [discussion: 665–7].

32. Konda VJ, Aslanian HR, Wallace MB, et al. First assessment of needle-based confocal laser endomicroscopy during EUS-FNA procedures of the pancreas (with videos). Gastrointest Endosc 2011;74:1049–60.

33. Napoleon B, Lemaistre AI, Pujol B, et al. A novel approach to the diagnosis of pancreatic serous cystadenoma: needle-based confocal laser endomicroscopy. Endoscopy 2015;47:26–32.

34. Nakai Y, Iwashita T, Park DH, et al. Diagnosis of pancreatic cysts: EUS-guided, through-the-needle confocal laser-induced endomicroscopy and cystoscopy trial: DETECT study. Gastrointest Endosc 2015;81:1204–14.

35. Barresi L, Crinò SF, Fabbri C, et al. Endoscopic ultrasound-through-the-needle biopsy in pancreatic cystic lesions: a multicenter study. Dig Endosc 2018. [Epub ahead of print].

36. Basar O, Yuksel O, Yang DJ, et al. Feasibility and safety of microforceps biopsy in the diagnosis of pancreatic cysts. Gastrointest Endosc 2018;88(1):79–86.

37. Wu J, Jiao Y, Dal Molin M, et al. Whole-exome sequencing of neoplastic cysts of the pancreas reveals recurrent mutations in components of ubiquitin-dependent pathways. Proc Natl Acad Sci U S A 2011;108:21188–93.

38. Singhi AD, Brand RE, Nikiforova MN, et al. American Gastroenterological Association guidelines are inaccurate in detecting pancreatic cysts with advanced neoplasia: a clinicopathologic study of 225 patients with supporting molecular data. Gastrointest Endosc 2016;83(6):1107–17.e2.

39. Hata T, Dal Molin M, Hong SM, et al. Predicting the grade of dysplasia of pancreatic cystic neoplasms using cyst fluid DNA methylation markers. Clin Cancer Res 2017;23:3935–44.

40. Hata T, Dal Molin M, Suenaga M, et al. Cyst fluid telomerase activity predicts the histologic grade of cystic neoplasms of the pancreas. Clin Cancer Res 2016;22: 5141–51.

41. Das KK, Xiao H, Geng X, et al. mAb Das-1 is specific for high-risk and malignant intraductal papillary mucinous neoplasm (IPMN). Gut 2014;63:1626–34.

Moving?

Make sure your subscription moves with you!

To notify us of your new address, find your **Clinics Account Number** (located on your mailing label above your name), and contact customer service at:

Email: **journalscustomerservice-usa@elsevier.com**

800-654-2452 (subscribers in the U.S. & Canada)
314-447-8871 (subscribers outside of the U.S. & Canada)

Fax number: **314-447-8029**

Elsevier Health Sciences Division
Subscription Customer Service
3251 Riverport Lane
Maryland Heights, MO 63043

*To ensure uninterrupted delivery of your subscription, please notify us at least 4 weeks in advance of move.

ELSEVIER

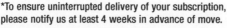

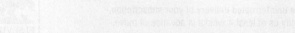

Printed and bound by CPI Group (UK) Ltd, Croydon, CR0 4YY

07/10/2024

01040506-0013